WHY FAST?

FOOD CONTROVERSIES

SERIES EDITOR: ANDREW F. SMITH

Everybody eats. Yet few understand the importance of food in our lives and the decisions we make each time we eat. The Food Controversies series probes problems created by the industrial food system and examines proposed alternatives.

Already published:

Fast Food: The Good, the Bad and the Hungry Andrew F. Smith
Food Adulteration and Food Fraud Jonathan Rees
In Defense of Processed Food Anastacia Marx de Salcedo
What's So Controversial about Genetically Modified Food? John T. Lang
What's the Matter with Meat? Katy Keiffer
Why Fast? The Pros and Cons of Restrictive Eating Christine Baumgarthuber
Why Waste Food? Andrew F. Smith

WHY FAST?

THE PROS AND CONS OF RESTRICTIVE EATING

CHRISTINE BAUMGARTHUBER

REAKTION BOOKS

To the memory of all the human and animal subjects of the starvation studies mentioned in this book

Published by

REAKTION BOOKS LTD
Unit 32, Waterside
44–48 Wharf Road
London N1 7UX, UK

www.reaktionbooks.co.uk

First published 2023

Printed and bound in Great Britain
by TJ Books Ltd, Padstow, Cornwall

A catalogue record for this book is available from the British Library
ISBN 978 1 78914 763 6

CONTENTS

1

A HUNGER FOR MORE: FASTING AND ITS PURPOSES FROM ANTIQUITY TO THE PRESENT

'Every day, try to be hungry and out of breath.'
– David Sinclair (Harvard geneticist)[1]

Fasting has been a part of my life, in one way or another, for as long as I can remember. Some of my earliest memories involve fasting. I lived in Vienna as a child, and my family regularly joined my grandparents for dinner. This was ever a delight for me because my Oma made excellent meals. We'd come to the table, each of us eager to tuck into sauerbraten or schnitzel that had been cooked to perfection – each of us eager, that is, except my grandfather. He'd hang back in the living room, seemingly impervious to the aromas reaching him. There, he would take off his shirt and arrange himself into a headstand.

I once asked my Opa, as he swayed in his inverted stance, why he didn't join the rest of us, who ate so heartily and well. From near the floor came a smile (which from my perspective, right-side up, looked more like a grimace), followed by words to the effect that forsaking home cooking for headstands cleared his mind and strengthened his body. Skipping a meal or two, he said, never hurt anyone. Indeed, he insisted that it had helped many people become healthier and stay that way.

Accustomed as I was to three meals daily, with snacks in between, I found myself both puzzled and fascinated by my Opa's answer. His notions made little sense to me – and the conviction with which he shared them, even less so.

Food in Abundance

My early confusion at the idea of fasting may perhaps be forgiven. I was a child of the 1980s, a decade which saw people in the West with more food to eat than ever before. By doing headstands during dinner time, then, my Opa turned his nose up at unprecedented abundance. Improved agricultural technology and government grain subsidies combined to create conditions in which food could be produced cheaper and faster than in decades past. Never before had citizens of Western countries had so many calories available to them at so low a cost. A comparison of household budgets across decades drives this fact home. More than 25 per cent of average Americans' income was spent on food in 1933, compared to only 10 per cent in 1997.[2]

Alongside the shrinking of household grocery expenses, food itself transformed over the years. The money that did still go into groceries was increasingly spent on foods like hamburgers, frozen pizza and chicken nuggets. Items of this kind are described as 'ultraprocessed', a designation that attaches to 'snacks, drinks, ready meals and many other products created mostly or entirely from substances extracted from foods or derived from food constituents with little if any intact food'. They are, in other words, submitted to manipulations by equipment not usually found in home kitchens. Such manipulation creates products with the chief virtues of convenience, addictive taste and, for the manufacturers, high profitability.[3] Sacrificed in the bargain are nutrition and a balanced diet: ultraprocessed foods encourage overeating like no other kind.

Despite their many pitfalls, ultraprocessed foods have experienced a growth in popularity over the decades. This growth appears like the mirror image of the trajectory of food costs generally in the same period. In 1938, the average Canadian, for example, had a diet that consisted of a little less than 25 per cent ultraprocessed food. By 2001, that had more than doubled, to nearly 55 per cent.[4] This single example suggests that ultraprocessed foods do live up to their virtues – convenience, especially. Ultraprocessed foods are seemingly everywhere. Over the decades we have gone from a relative absence of such foods to a land not so much of milk and honey, but certainly of candy bars, sausage sticks and doughnuts.

Ultraprocessed foods have ushered us into a fool's paradise. The average individual of the late twentieth century thought about food more than two hundred times a day.[5] A great many of these thoughts became deeds: in the closing years of the 1990s, snacks alone made up one-fourth of the average American child's daily diet.[6] Adults in the early twenty-first century manage no better. Many of them eat four times a day or more.[7] Young folks today no longer think in terms of daily meals. They think in terms of 'eating events', which, as you may suppose, happen early and often.[8]

How did it come to pass that people in the West went from more or less regular mealtimes (if they were lucky) to eating events crowding their waking hours? It's a question with no simple answer. Yet for some insight we may consider modern marketing. Ultraprocessed food is overwhelmingly the product of huge corporations. Their advertising of these products has contributed to an 'obesogenic' environment – that is, an environment that encourages overeating to ruinous physical effect. Television, one of the more dominant features of this environment, abounds with advertisements that encourage us to eat, and the very act of viewing it fosters long bouts of inactivity. Music does its part, as well; the faster a song's beat, in fact, the faster we shovel in the snacks. Many of us do a lot of work on computers. Work done this way widens our appetites by stimulating our bodies to produce the hormone cortisol. If that work is often stressful, our cortisol levels only increase further.[9] So vast has the obesogenic environment grown that it has become increasingly difficult to find refuge from the summons to eat and eat and then eat some more.

My First Fast

It has come to pass that we live, work, play and sleep (or try to) in an environment that seduces us to eat poorly and often. This being so, what possible place could fasting have in this environment? A version of this question occupied me in my early thirties when I attempted my own fast. Perhaps I was inspired in part by the memory of my Opa, since deceased. I found encouragement when I stumbled upon a second-hand copy of *How to Keep Slim, Healthy, and Young with Juice Fasting*, a manual published in 1971 by the

Finnish health guru Paavo Airola. From its well-thumbed pages chirped assurances that a regimen of raw juices, if faithfully followed, would prove revolutionary. It would help me to wring impurities from my tissues and peel away the consequences of neglectful past eating habits. It would deliver me, in the author's words, to 'total rejuvenation of all the functions of the body'.[10]

The sweeping claims as to fasting's many benefits led me to further research. I sought to substantiate Airola's programme with findings in medical literature. The literature was either silent on Airola's manual or hostile to it; the health guru was deemed a quack in many quarters. The medical literature did, however, present a host of health benefits that fasting provides, supported by scientific investigation. The list was impressive and included improved insulin resistance, the reversal of metabolic syndrome (a group of conditions that place one at risk of developing type 2 diabetes) and increased cognitive function, not to mention reduced blood pressure, lowered heart rate, improved long- and short-term memory and weight loss, among other benefits.

These findings were music to my ears. It wasn't that I suffered anything that fasting could reverse. I just figured that by taking up fasting while still young and healthy I could head off anything that I might have needed to reverse later in life – the proverbial ounce of prevention, pound of cure. To this end, I gathered the ingredients for my maiden fast.

It wasn't Airola's juice fast, as it happened. I opted, rather, for a drink altogether unlikely. It consisted of B-grade maple syrup, lemon juice, cayenne pepper and spring water. These I mixed in a shaker bottle and took to work. I'd named Friday as my fasting day, and sipped my concoction throughout it. I fended off hunger pangs by imagining the healing magic the fast was working on my body, which until that point had metabolized food daily for some three decades.

I wish I could claim that my resolve lasted so long. It crumbled after two weeks. My stomach growled and growled. Dizziness washed over me at odd times and without warning. Snacks dumped on the table in the office break room worked on me like catnip. And it didn't help that my fasting-day drink had a flavour somewhere between fiery hot marinade and bathroom cleanser. My willpower sapped, I found myself absorbed by the obesogenic day-to-day once again. And I found myself asking, once more, why fast?

Indeed, given its difficulty, why should we fast? That's the question this book seeks to answer. But please understand that none of the information in it should be construed as medical advice. The decision to fast ought not to be made lightly. I hope that this stroll through fasting's history will bring you closer to a sense of whether the practice is right for you.

Our stroll will begin with early inquiries into the act of eating – the need for it and the consequences of forgoing it. We'll then see how the fruits of these inquiries led to innovations in weight-loss diets and greater understanding of fasting's many health benefits. Along with those benefits come certain dangers; we'll consider these as well. We'll end with a look at the various technological enhancements brought to the practice of fasting, which has surged in popularity in recent years. Once we're through, you will, I hope, have been immersed in the subject fully enough to arrive at a decision as to whether fasting offers more attractive rewards than the gustatory temptations dangled before you.

Fasting or Starvation?

It makes sense at the outset to distinguish fasting from starvation. Though experience of the first can certainly feel like the second, there is a distinction. It's reflected in their etymology: 'starve' comes from the German verb *sterben*, which means 'to die', and today we associate starvation with death through lack of food. But the twentieth-century poet and scholar John Ciardi made the interesting observation that the word only recently came to acquire this meaning. 'In Chaucer's day,' he writes, '"sterven" – from the Anglo Saxon steorfan . . . meant any slow death, as by exposure, torture, hunger, or thirst.'[11] Towns were 'starved out' as a means of forcing their surrender.[12] And since this usually meant, for the most part, denying the townsfolk food, the word came to denote only this.

'Fast', meanwhile, derives from the Old German *fest*, which means to remain solid or fixed – to 'hold something fast', for example. The word was used to describe a way of observing a period of abstinence. And here we see the difference between fasting and starving. Fasting is active, a stubborn exercise of will. Think of a wan anchorite refusing even a communion wafer, or a dieter grimly sipping grapefruit juice for days on end. Starvation, on the other hand, is passive, a punishment inflicted by hostile armies, fickle weather and calloused plutocrats. 'After our Lord was baptized, he fasted,' reads the Anglo-Saxon *Blickling Homilies* of 971 CE – the earliest evidence we have of an English use of the word. Were he to have been denied food, he would have starved.

Sometimes, however, the distinctions blur. A fast may be carried to the point of death, as it is in fatal anorexia cases. Yet in such cases the fasters have exercised their will, captive though it may have been to an unhealthy fixation.

Fasting as a Spiritual Practice

Many of us think of fasting as first and foremost a spiritual practice. And for millennia that is what it was. Certain indigenous groups in Central and North America, for example, saw fasting as a way to connect with the divine. Ethnographic studies in the 1920s and '30s showed that the Tepecano people of Mexico fasted as a way of bringing relief to a village cursed with sickness and death. The act was also relied upon as a way of influencing happy outcomes in pursuits as diverse as planting corn, hunting deer and building homes.[13]

The Omaha people of northern Nebraska practised fasting before recounting sacred tales. The Mandan of North Dakota fasted before worship.[14] The Mandan people's neighbours to the west, the Crow, had a legend that told of a young man of their tribe who fasted so he could glimpse 'the country where the birds lived'. His sacrifice found purchase, for on 'the fourth day he fasted a meadow lark came and wanted to adopt him'.[15]

Fasting also played a role in mustering spirit of a different kind – namely, that needed for waging war and playing competitive sport. Warriors of the Creek people, originally of the American southeast, steeled themselves for the warpath by drinking a mysterious elixir they called 'the black drink', an act which they followed with a three-day fast lest 'the power of their purifying . . . physic' fail.[16] A stickball game invented by the Creek people's neighbours, the Choctaws, required contestants to fast prior to the game, and they were prohibited from eating until the contest was completed the following day.[17]

In other parts of the world, fasting became the speciality of a priest class who refined the practice into a drawn-out flirtation with death. And this flirtation with death was also with whatever – or whoever – lay beyond death. The priests of Babylonia, a region in present-day Iraq first settled in the fourth millennium BCE, presided over penitential fasts intended to calm an angry god. In ancient Egypt priests fasted before entering their temples, and pharaohs fasted before making decisions. Fasting was said to clear the mind and body, intensifying the effects of spells and prayers and offering elevation to the heavenly realm.

It is perhaps this impulse towards the otherworldly that kept fasting, in its most extreme form, from the perception of simply suicide by starvation. Fasters wished to attain greater meaning and fulfilment than they could find in their corporeal lives. There prevailed the belief that the practice restored its practitioners from a fallen state to one of blessedness, of grace.

Fasting and Major Religions

This line of thinking can be seen in all the major religions. The Jews fasted to please and seek forgiveness from God, as King David fasted in atonement for his dalliance with Bathsheba, which had caused him to betray his loyal general Uriah. Fasting remains an important practice in modern Judaism. Yom Kippur, a day of atonement and the most important holiday in the Jewish faith, sees practitioners going without food from sundown to sundown, a period of about 25 hours. And fasts from sundown to sunrise are a feature of more minor fasting days.

For Muslims fasting is one of the Five Pillars of Islam. During Ramadan, a period that celebrates the first revelation of the Qur'an to Mohammed, Muslims are prohibited from eating from dawn to dusk. The Ramadan fast, known as *sawm*, serves to remind them of their utter reliance on Allah for the goods of this life, and it recalls to them their obligation to the vulnerable and less fortunate members of their spiritual community.[18]

Adherents of Hinduism fast for several reasons. The practice is said to cleanse body and mind, as well as any negative energy that might taint an auspicious occasion. It plays a crucial role in sacraments, festivals and holidays. Fasting is said to bring the devoted faster to a transcendent awareness of the gods.[19] So populous is the Hindu pantheon that different days of the week are assigned to fasting in worship of a particular deity. Worshippers of Shiva fast on Monday, worshippers of Vishnu on Thursday. Tuesday belongs to no one god; worshippers of any could fast if they so liked, and Tuesday therefore remains a popular fast day in contemporary India.

Fasting in Buddhism served a purpose that was elegantly simple in contrast. The practice gained traction because the Buddha himself, Siddhartha Gautama (fifth century BCE), engaged in it. To this end, Buddhist monks and nuns eat nothing after their noon meal. In this they follow their paragon's example. 'Not eating a meal in the evening,' the Buddha said, meant 'I, monks, am aware of good health and of being without illness and of buoyancy and strength and living in comfort.'[20] Yet he disapproved of outright starvation. Having once submitted himself to a period of extreme fasting, he concluded that the path to enlightenment lay through a 'middle way' between inanition and gluttony.

Christians, however, saw no such middle way. They embroidered upon and refined fasting, taking it to exquisite extremes. In the desert wastes of Egypt and Syria, Christian monks of the first few centuries of the common era subsisted on raw pulses and herbs steeped in water to achieve divine insight. Service to the soul, which they believed to partake of special celestial substance, meant subduing and mortifying its material vessel, the body. Through his early and middle twenties the hermit Hilarion (291–371), for example, ate nothing but lentils soaked in cold water. He followed this diet with several others in succession: bread, salt and water; wild herbs and roots; and vegetables and barley bread. By the time Hilarion was 63 years old, his enfeebled stomach could handle only a broth of herbs and meal taken daily at sunset. He believed that simple foods, which he was certain must have been enjoyed in Eden, brought him closer to God.[21]

As the centuries passed, people continued to seek close-ness to God through fasting – though it often proved fatal. St Catherine of Siena (1347–1380), known for her abstinence, took her claim to fame to new heights in her early thirties by protesting that she could no longer eat anything at all. She often prayed that she might, for people thought her a witch whom demons fed at night, to no avail. She continued her fast and soon became paralysed, dying at age 33. St Marie of Oignies (1177–1213) was another fatal faster. She so hated the smell of food that she reportedly put off meal-taking for as long as 35 days. Here and there, she would nibble the odd tidbit. But soon she found even this revolting, and so stopped eating altogether. Like Catherine, Marie was in her thirties when she died.

In these examples of spiritual austerity we see that fasting does not differ much from starvation. We may well wonder whether this cultivation of extreme fasting left an impression in Western minds, with some viewing the practice as an inherently unpleasant and unsound exercise. As we will see, however, fasting can assume many forms, some more pleasant than others. The more extreme examples of fasting merely demonstrate the adaptable nature of the human body. Indeed, saints and sinners alike could not have undertaken such extreme fasts had their bodies been unable to endure long periods of starvation. Such endurance owed to certain biological adaptations.

What Happens When We Eat

Now that we have an idea of what fasting means etymologically, we can turn our sights to what it means biologically. But before we discuss what happens when we fast, let's look at what happens when we eat.

When it comes to eating, we do what our bodies require – but we do it for pleasure. This fact sometimes makes us forget just how dependent we are on fairly regular nourishment. 'Normal life', write physicians Maurice Shils and Moshe Shike, 'may be defined as the conversion of energy to perform meaningful work at an acceptable metabolic cost.'[22] Our bodies are like our bank accounts. You want neither to overdraw funds nor to accumulate so much in any one account that it becomes a liability. Like sound personal finance, sound health depends on maintaining a balance.

Our bodies do a deft job of processing everything we 'deposit'. Salad, sundae and salami alike become broken down into the basic constituents for supplying energy and growing and repairing tissues and bone. The breaking down begins with the first bite. As we chew, enzymes in our saliva break down starches. Digestion continues in our stomach as the food mixes with acids and more enzymes. In our small intestine, bile from our liver breaks up fat globules. The glands of our pancreas and intestine secrete enzymes that act on specific molecules, reducing carbohydrates to simple sugars, proteins to amino acids and fat into glycerol and fatty acids – all of which are absorbed into the bloodstream through the intestinal walls. Fibre and other indigestible matter move to our large intestine, where water and ions are reabsorbed. The rest? Well, that's deposited elsewhere.

The job of processing whatever we deposit in our bodies happens at one rate or another depending on our individual condition and constitution. We often talk of having a fast or slow metabolism. But what does that mean? 'Metabolism' is a blanket term that describes two processes. The first process is catabolism. This is the process by which our body extracts energy for fuelling itself. The second process is anabolism. This is the process by which our body obtains the organic material it needs for repairing itself. Both processes go on in digestion. When we concern ourselves with the question of whether our metabolism is slow or fast, then, we have in mind the rate at which our body completes the processes of catabolism and anabolism.[23]

Most discussions of metabolism centre on calories. A calorie is simply a measure of the amount of energy required to raise the temperature of one gram of water by one degree centigrade.[24] Caloric energy is housed in fat, protein and carbohydrates – the macronutrients for sustaining life. (Equally essential micronutrients exist as well, as do smaller nutrient categories, such as vitamins and minerals.) If you skimp on any of these macronutrients long enough, you'll suffer serious consequences. Carbohydrates are the most plentiful (and some say the most savoury) among the biological molecules that supply us with calories. Fats, on the other hand, are the most plentiful in calories themselves: nine per gram to carbohydrates' four. For their part, proteins supply four calories per gram, though our bodies have a tougher time accessing these calories.

Whatever the respective virtues or drawbacks of fat, protein and carbohydrates, our bodies nevertheless need all three of these macronutrients, and a number of micronutrients, for survival. Yet it turns out certain parts of our body are less ecumenical, nutritionally speaking, than others. Our brain, for example, favours carbohydrates – and a specific carbohydrate at that. That carbohydrate is glucose, a simple sugar. For our brain, no other nutrient will do in most cases (the exception we'll discuss below). The rest of our tissues and organs, meanwhile, content themselves equally with fatty acids. Yet our brain must have the nutrient it demands, so the rest of our body bends to the task of ensuring an ample supply. Protein, fat and carbohydrate alike are rendered into glucose by one bodily process or another. Because the rest of our body parts depend on the brain in order to function, they ensure it gets fed – even in times of caloric dearth. Even if we should diet or fast, the brain demands its due feeding of glucose.

What Happens When We Fast?

Let's say you decide to skip dinner. Once you've completely digested your lunch, a process which takes a few hours, you experience a drop in your levels of insulin, a hormone responsible for regulating the amount of glucose in your blood. In response to the drop in insulin, three other hormones – cortisol, glucagon and epinephrine – flood in to the rescue. These are all catabolic hormones, meaning they help our body extract energy for fuelling itself. Cortisol, glucagon and epinephrine work together to help your liver convert fatty and amino acids into glucose.[25] It is through this process that your body maintains homeostasis of blood sugar levels. This process is known as gluconeogenesis, and it works to ensure that your brain can continue to function.[26]

Suppose now that you extend your abstention to include the following day's breakfast and lunch. Your body responds to the additional meals missed by dipping into its fat stores. Go without eating for a few more days and your body moves on from the fat stores it has exhausted to relying on muscle tissue for energy. How long you can continue in this state depends on the fat and muscle reserves you had at the outset. In a given day, fasting individuals of average size might burn 1,800 calories derived from 75 grams (2.6 oz) of skeletal muscle protein and 160 grams (5.6 oz) of triglycerides from fat. Under the right conditions (that is, suffering no additional trauma or deprivation in the form of exposure to extreme temperatures and other conditions), they can survive about eighty days without food.[27] You really would not want your body eating muscle, however; consumed in the bargain may be the most important muscle of all, your heart. At any rate, once muscle tissue begins to be consumed, starvation and death soon follow.

Starvation Is in Our Genes

The chapters to follow contain much more discussion of starvation's physical effects. It suffices here to say that our body's ability to survive eighty days without food points to the fact that we as a species have lived with dearth longer than we have lived with abundance. The spectre of starvation has stalked humanity for millennia. 'Hunger, or the fear of it, has always played a major role in determining the actions and the attitudes of man,' wrote the American physiologist Ancel Keys in 1950. 'In every age and every land people have starved.'[28] Such close familiarity with starvation encoded in our genes the means for surviving it.

The human genotype, or collection of inherited traits and characteristics, is believed to have evolved between 600,000 and 25,000 BCE. During this period, our efforts at hunting and gathering met with uneven success.[29] Over half our hunter-gatherer ancestors' diet came from animal sources, a dependence accompanied by all the attendant uncertainty of a hunt's outcome. When a hunt came up empty, days without food would follow. Our ancient ancestors expected these bouts of dearth, and even accepted them as inevitable. (In truth these bouts were fewer than those that visited later sedentary agricultural communities.) Over time their bodies learned to cope with these periods of fasting, gaining an ability to store fat more readily and use more efficiently any nutrients that were on hand. In times of plenty they feasted. In times of want they fasted – easy of mind, if not enthusiastically.

An accommodation to bouts of hunger survived into recorded history. Exemplary of this were the Indigenous groups of colonial New England (c. 1621–91). An early settler by the name of Samuel Lee observed that '10 times in 24 houres' the tribespeople (Wampanoag, most likely) would eat after the successful slaying of 'a beare or a deere'.[30] By the same token, Lee noted, they would be 'very patient in fasting, & will gird in their bellies till they meet with food'.[31]

Their patience perhaps found support in an understanding that it was as nature ordained. And, indeed, their long bouts of hunger served the tribe by reducing fertility during those periods – a natural form of population control, which helped to ensure that the tribe never strained available resources.

Could we living today meet long bouts of hunger with equal acceptance? Something of an answer to this question came in 2011, when researchers led an eleven-person group on a ten-day trip through the Pyrenees, the range of mountains that divides France and Spain. The purpose of the trek was to have the participants live for a short while like hunter-gatherers. The group followed strict rules in pursuit of maximum fidelity to the hunter-gatherer experience. Drinking could take place only whenever they came across watering holes, despite the distance separating one from the next sometimes being as great as 48 kilometres (30 mi.); and any eating could take place only twice a day, and only of animals the participants had hunted, killed and dressed themselves. Hunger and thirst gripped the participants through the trek's first three days. By its seventh day, they all wanted to go home, claiming exhaustion. By its end, however, most of them reported that they 'enjoyed the trip and recognized the benefits by feeling healthier' and that they had recovered 'from Western stressful life'.[32] They had grown used to going a long time without anything to eat or drink – and believed themselves better for it.

Fasting in the Animal Kingdom

The ability to fast even under the most trying circumstances is something humans share with many living creatures. It exists in unicellular *Saccharomyces cerevisiae*, the yeast in beer and bread. (Indeed, *S. cerevisiae* not only bears fasting but in fact benefits from it, the experience doubling its lifespan.) Larger creatures likewise have this ability. Birds fast in their migratory flights, during which they sustain their highest metabolic rate as they wing their way across oceans and continents. Bar-tailed godwits, for example, fast through some two hundred hours of flight from Alaska to New Zealand. Seal pups learn how to fast early in life. Weaned abruptly when their mother goes to sea in search of food, they go without eating for weeks. Salmon fast when they migrate, losing up to 80 per cent of their body weight.[33] Even the tiniest animals fast. Cave-dwelling newts may go without food for several years, an ability which may make them the vertebrates that are best adapted to fasting conditions.[34] And the diminutive golden spiny mouse, which lives in the vast arid deserts of West Asia, can reduce its metabolism and oxygen intake to endure long stretches of privation.[35]

Perhaps the most impressive animal faster of all is the male emperor penguin. He keeps a lonely and foodless winter vigil over a single egg on the Antarctic sea ice, enduring winds of 200 kilometres per hour (125 mph) and temperatures of -50°C (-58.0°F) for his trouble. To prepare for his fast he spends the preceding months scouring the ocean for food, gaining about 113 grams (4 oz) of fat daily. The fat is deposited in the body so quickly that it resembles, chemically speaking, the creatures from which it came.[36] Extract a lump of it and you would be hard pressed to say whether it came from a penguin or the silverfish, krill or squid he had dined on just hours before. (The emperor penguin must take care that he avoids gaining too much weight, however, lest he find himself slow, succulent prey to leopard seals and orcas.)

Once the penguin has properly fattened himself, he swims home to his nest, where he will stay for the next four months. He arrives home already in a fasting state, his now-ample fat stores supplying his body with energy. Weight melts from his frame as the days and weeks pass. All the while, he remains seated above his egg, moving only when necessary. Near his vigil's end, his fat stores exhausted, muscle tissue has become his body's source of energy. His weight loss speeds up; because his muscles' energy yield is at least nine times lower than the yield from his fat, more muscle tissue is consumed to keep his body adequately supplied.[37]

Other creatures in the animal kingdom pay the ultimate price. The fast of the giant deep-sea octopus *Graneledone boreopacifica* stands as an example. In the frigid depths of the ocean, the female octopus lays a clutch of 50 to 75 eggs, over which she drapes her strongly textured, ruby-purple mantle and her long, sinewy arms. She remains in the position for her eggs' entire four-year gestation period, consuming her energy stores all the while. As her stores become depleted, her robust and colourful skin turns a sickly white. Her eyes, once as shiny as sea glass, cloud and sink into her waning flesh. Her skin smooths and slackens. Her tentacles wither. 'The same octopus [clings] to the vertical rock wall, arms curled, covering her eggs,' notes one researcher who studies

Graneledone boreopacifica. Shrimp and crabs – her favourite foods – swirl and scuttle about her. Yet she makes no attempt at catching them. Rather, she brushes them aside, as though afraid they would tempt her from her sole duty. At the end of the fourth year the mother vanishes, likely dead. All that remains of her vigil are bits of the eggs she had guarded so doggedly.[38]

The emperor penguin and the deep-sea octopus offer but two examples of fasting in the animal kingdom. They highlight fasting's utility in that realm: namely, to conserve energy for survival and reproduction. The ability to fast enjoyed by us human beings may have similar roots, but it is also much more personal, thanks to our ability to think and reflect. Starvation is a hunger condition thrust upon on us, usually after food stores run out or are destroyed. When we thrust that hunger condition on ourselves by our own free will, be it for greater spiritual awareness, health or longevity, we have crossed from starvation to fasting. In this way fasting becomes a seemingly paradoxical feat: both ensconcing us in physical existence and transcending it.

Fasting for any of those purposes comes to seem strange in an obesogenic environment such as ours in the West. The chapters to follow endeavour to remove this strangeness and reacquaint us with the virtues of fasting, as well as its perils. Yet before such a reacquaintance can happen, we must first consider human nutrition – specifically, how the latter became an object of study and what findings this study uncovered.

2

FOOD FOR THOUGHT: FASTING THROUGH THE AGES

'I entered into the joyous frenzy of hunger. I was empty and free from pain, and I gave free rein to my thoughts.' – Knut Hamsun, *Hunger* (1890)[1]

September and October 2003 saw unusually large numbers of people gather throughout the day in London's Potters Field Park, which sits on the southern bank of the river Thames. The parkgoers were observably animated, commenting and pointing as they directed their gazes skyward at a most novel sight: a Plexiglas box resembling an aquarium, some 9 metres (30 ft) over their heads and held in place by cables and guy wires; and in this box, a living man, sometimes standing, sometimes reclining on some bedding.

The man in the box was David Blaine, a young magician who vaulted to stardom in the late 1990s with his postmodern takes on the magician's television special, *Street Magic* and *Magic Man*. Adept at card tricks and illusions, Blaine was also an accomplished endurance artist. He had arranged to be buried alive for a week on one occasion and encased in ice for nearly three days on another. These stunts he followed with what he framed as an update of the early Christian stylites' ascetic practice, perching himself atop a tall pillar in New York City and remaining there for some 35 hours.

The state of suspended confinement in the Plexiglas box above London in 2003 – *Above the Below*, as he named it – represented the latest stage of this second aspect of his career. Hoisted aloft on 5 September, for 44 days he dangled, his only supplies diapers, a journal and pen, some lip balm and a rubber tube for delivering water.

While some spectators cheered him on, others tempted him with food, either by throwing it at his box, or, in one instance, airlifting it on a remote-controlled helicopter. One diabolical onlooker even tried to clip his tube.

On the morning of 19 October, Blaine signalled that he had reached his limit. Exhausted, lighter by some 23 kilograms (50 lb) and yet triumphant, he emerged, announcing, 'This has been one of the most important experiences of my life.'[2] Then he broke into tears. When later asked why he had put himself through the ordeal, he answered, 'I was obsessed with the idea of fasting and isolation.'[3] Onlookers of a darker cast of mind were no doubt obsessed with the idea of a man publicly starving himself to death.

A Body's Inner Fire

The human body may endure weeks, even months, of starvation. But it took human minds millennia to develop an understanding beyond starvation's effects to a more nuanced understanding of its processes. In the following pages we will trace the history of that understanding. Much of the evidence cited today for fasting – the beneficial health and weight loss effects – were discoveries made over millennia. And each one of these discoveries advanced our knowledge of the surprising and seemingly miraculous workings of the body.

Our first inklings as to the need for food likely came when we began to wonder about two phenomena we had observed in ourselves: the warmth of our bodies, and the difficulty we had in maintaining this warmth. Our earliest ancestors likely noticed that such difficulty grew when they themselves grew hungry, and that it did so despite warm furs to wear and roaring fires to sit by. A fire within also needed stoking, it seemed to them, and meats, nuts and berries stoked it best. Whenever the inner fire ebbed, the form housing it cooled, growing thin and weak in the bargain. Allowed to ebb too long, the fire would finally go out.

The body's inner fire and its connection to nutrition were preoccupations in the classical age, which fell roughly between the 8th century BCE and the 6th century CE. (We will explore how these ideas first developed in the East in the next chapter.) 'Growing creatures have the most innate heat,' observed ancient Greek physician Hippocrates (460–375 BCE), 'and it is for this reason they need the most food, deprived of which their body pines away.'[4] The philosopher Aristotle (384–322 BCE) went further, linking the connection between heat and nourishment to the other markers of life: thinking, perception, local movement and rest, appetite, growth and, finally, decay.[5]

These towering figures of the classical age developed elaborate theories as to how this vital flame stayed alive and, in turn, kept the human body alive. It burned in the heart, they claimed, fuelled by the stomach as the latter digested food. 'It is out of food rather than out of the air that we see heat developed,' Aristotle wrote. This heat, in turn, aided digestion by converting – or 'concocting', as he called the process – food in the stomach into the stuff that made for more blood, semen and other bodily fluids, as well as flesh, bone and other body parts.[6] The converting of fluids and flesh from food bound every individual to a shared necessity. The elderly required less food for their 'concocting' than the young. But however great or slight the need, if there was not any food at all to feed it, death would come for individuals of any age sooner or later.

Such reasoning strikes present-day ears as flawed (not to mention anatomically incorrect). Unlike individuals who lived in classical antiquity, we benefit from many subsequent years of investigation aided with increasingly sophisticated instruments. Yet Aristotle, Hippocrates and their fellow ancients deserve credit for developing some of the earliest theories aimed at anchoring bodily processes in the natural realm. Before them, superstition dominated the thinking of ordinary men and women when it came to just about every facet of reality, alimentation included. For these people, reality unfolded from moment to moment according to the activities of gods and other powers. The leading thinkers of classical antiquity took the first steps forwards by doubting the conventional view. And they made their second step when they drew on their scepticism to elaborate a competing view, the hallmarks of which rested on the physical elements of air, earth, fire and water. These constituent elements of every part of the universe were determined also to constitute human individuals, who existed as microcosms of the universe. This correspondence between the universe and its many microcosms underpinned the idea that the former and the latter were equally subject to natural laws. One such law demanded that the fire of life must have fuel to remain lit; in human microcosms this happened by eating food.

Yet governmental laws sometimes prevented Aristotle, Hippocrates and their ilk from doing much in the way of validating natural laws. Dissection of human bodies was illegal in ancient Greece. This prohibition precluded any hands-on investigations aimed at finding physical evidence in support of the theoretical universe–humanity correspondence. One classical figure, however, would flout the prohibition, vivisecting criminals and recording his findings. He was the anatomist Erasistratus (304–250 BCE), and he wrote on medical topics ranging from the mechanisms of blood circulation to the nature of nerves that traverse the brain. Later founding a school of anatomy in the Egyptian city of Alexandria, Erasistratus developed theories that were closer to the reality of biological processes of the human body – so much closer, in fact, that his investigations eventually earned him recognition as the founder of physiology.[7]

The process of digestion was of particular interest to Erasistratus. He didn't much care for Hippocrates' take on it; the latter's notions of concoction and transmutation struck him as too theoretical. Intent on pulling an explanation of digestion down from the rare air of the theoretical and planting it in the rich earth of empiricism, Erasistratus devised an experiment. His experimental subjects were birds. Before he fed them, he weighed them, and then he weighed them a second time after they fed. He also weighed them after they defecated (or 'eliminated'), placing droppings and their sources in a scale together. He noticed that although the birds weighed less after elimination, the elimination did not account for all the weight lost. In fact, they were lighter than their pre-elimination weight minus the weight of their faeces.

Erasistratus' explanation for the greater-than-expected lightness has been lost to history, thanks to the burning of the Great Library of Alexandria in 391 CE. (Modern science suggests that the lightness was due to fluid lost through respiration, among other things.) Most of his writings were consumed in the fire. The smattering of his work that has been left to us survived as fragments cited in the work of later physicians and philosophers. One such physician was Galen (129–c. 216 CE), a towering figure in ancient medicine whose influence would continue to be felt well into the early modern period.

Like Erasistratus, Galen championed hands-on examination. In service to this principle, he rooted around inside fallen gladiators and dead pigs to discover the internal mechanisms of nutrition. Food began digesting in the stomach, Galen found. It was then expelled through the pylorus – a cone-shaped anatomical structure that joins the stomach to the small intestine – by way of an involuntary relaxation and constriction of the digestive tract, an action known as gastric peristalsis. Because he lived in a time well before the advent of biochemistry, however, his observations quickly ceded to speculation. He imagined that food worked its way through the alimentary tract, transforming into nutriment as it did so. In its new form it flowed to various parts of the body.

Nutrition, then, was this action of nutriment 'being worked up into' the body's every reach, Galen claimed.[8] The cause of the flow he termed 'the nutritive faculty'.[9] Galen presented the life animating the human form in analogies that would have struck his predecessor Aristotle as familiar. He wrote that the body was akin to a lamp: blood served as its oil; the heart, its wick. The lungs, he added, worked as 'an instrument which conveys motion'.[10] He understood the motion conveyed by them to cool the heart, thus regulating it.

Not much motion in terms of advancement beyond Galen's ideas would be witnessed for another 1,300 years. Yet from antiquity through those intervening centuries much was done with some of the fundamental insights that were established early on. Keystones of this knowledge were that nutrition was the body's way of warming and repairing itself; that without food to fuel it the body could perform neither warming nor repairing, to fatal consequence; and that the progression towards that consequence was starvation. On these simple insights would be built a complex science of diet and its effect on health – a science known as dietetics. Indeed, much of the advice we still follow today comes from dietetic prescriptions developed millennia ago, such as eating in moderation, avoiding 'heavy' foods – meat and cheese, for example – and fasting when overweight or ill.

Some prescriptions later revealed themselves as wrong, even disastrously so. The diet that Hippocrates recommended for treating diabetes, for example, consisted of milk, cereals, starch, groats and gruels – all dishes that would bring on insulin shock. The hit-or-miss quality of classical dietetics owed to gaps in knowledge about nutrition and metabolism, as we saw above with Galen. It would take until the Renaissance for these gaps to begin to be filled. And we may thank an eccentric Swiss physician for undertaking a good deal of the spadework.

Renaissance Thinkers

That eccentric Swiss individual was Philippus Aureolus Theophrastus Bombastus von Hohenheim (1493–1541), remembered as Paracelsus, the less daunting pseudonym he later adopted. Born to a respectable middle-class family residing in the Swiss town of Einsiedeln, as a young man Paracelsus preferred the company of alchemists and barbers to that of scholars. He loved knowledge of all kinds except the kind touted by traditional academics in the universities he despised. He sniffed at such institutions, seeing them as productive of nothing but, as he put it, 'so many high asses'.[11] Even greater contempt he reserved for the ancient Greek and Roman authorities (Hippocrates, Aristotle and Galen, among others) revered by those high asses. So great was his contempt, in fact, that he cursed and denounced those classical thinkers and burned their works in public. The gesture proved symbolic, for it was Paracelsus' desire that a new science rise from the ashes of past learning – a new science that better reflected the realities of the natural world.

What Paracelsus' embryonic new science may initially have lacked in rigour and systematicity, it made up for in eclecticism. In his idiosyncratic way, Paracelsus studied everything from metallurgy and alchemy to herbalism. He worked for a time in the mines of southern Austria, where he watched with rapt attention the transformation of metal from solid to liquid in smelting vats.[12] The experience left him convinced that chemicals were the fundamental constituents of the world and everything in it. In service to this conviction, he tossed into his alembic items – fruit, wood, flowers, leaves – whose essences he believed to harm or help people's health. The alembic did the work of distilling these essences, and from them Paracelsus concocted various elixirs. His experiments in this area led him to the further conviction that nature held the cure for every disease afflicting humanity. The trick lay in employing the proper chemical methods for drawing out the proper healing essences. In coaxing healing secrets from the bosom of nature with the help of his alembics and retorts, Paracelsus became the father of pharmacology.

Paracelsus' preoccupation with essences led him down other avenues of inquiry into human health. 'In everything there is an essence and a poison,' Paracelsus wrote, defining essence in this context as 'that which preserves man' and poison as 'that which produces illness'.[13] Even food was of this dual substance. Paracelsus went on to claim that 'every animal has a food adapted to it.'[14] How an animal managed to extract the essence and avoid injury from the poison in its food depended on the 'alchemist' that resided in its stomach. This alchemist, properly known as the 'Archaeus' – and wholly of Paracelsus' invention – was a sort of directing force or spirit, and it divided wholesome substances in food from unwholesome.[15] If the Archaeus was doing its work well, high health followed. Poor health, meanwhile, indicated that the Archaeus itself had somehow become incapacitated.[16]

However outré Paracelsus' thinking seems to modern minds, it nonetheless supplied the preliminary concepts for moving beyond sclerotic theories that had held sway for centuries. And it opened the door to a new way of understanding the body and its nutritional needs.[17] Experiment, observation, experience, the natural sciences – Paracelsus valued them all, and in valuing them showed himself an early exponent of what would coalesce as textbook scientific inquiry in the West.

Paracelsus was not alone in devising new ways of thinking about the workings of the human body. Around the same time, an amiable physician with the delightful name of Santorio Santorio (1561–1636) toiled at fathoming the mysteries of metabolism. Santorio devised a thermometer to measure body heat and an ingenious weighing chair to measure a particular kind of weight loss. Such weight loss happened when a fasting individual had neither broken his fast nor moved his bowels. Santorio named this 'insensible perspiration', and he had an idea that it had something to do with someone's state of health.[18] He believed, as he wrote, that 'all bad illnesses usually originate from a smaller or larger perspiration than is proper.'[19] Santorio made himself the subject in an experiment to test his theory. He prepared a meal and weighed it. He then sat in his special chair to weigh himself. After weighing himself, he ate his meal while still seated in the chair, taking bite after bite until his chair dipped lower. When this happened, he ended his meal. After his meal made its journey through him, he weighed the resulting waste products. Urine and faeces together weighed less than the meal, he found. The result recalled the experiments made centuries earlier by Erasistratus on his birds.

It may seem a madness, all this weighing. But method did lay behind it. Santorio's experiments introduced the idea of quantitative research into physiology, the tenets of which he elaborated in a series of aphorisms he composed in (where else!) his weighing chair.[20] The good doctor claimed, through his careful measurements, to have gathered ample proof of insensible perspiration.[21] More importantly, however, Santorio modelled how one might learn more about the human body and its processes through observation and quantifiable data.

Experiments proliferated in the age ushered in by Paracelsus and Santorio, as did investigations into phenomena that had seemed wholly divine just a century prior. Physicians who followed in the latter men's footsteps were presented with a great boon that helped them to venture beyond the mechanics of nutrition to the mechanics of starvation. The boon came in the form of several fasting women, so-called 'miraculous maids', who came on to the scene in the sixteenth century.

One important document of the study of fasting women, published by the Dutch physician Johann Weyer in 1577, recounted the case of Elizabeth Barton (1506–1534). Barton earned notoriety, along with the moniker 'the Maid of Kent', for her diet, what there was of it. It purportedly consisted of communion wafers and nothing besides. And they were no ordinary wafers, unlike those dispensed by priests during a Catholic liturgy. Rather, they dropped from heaven, or so the reaper of that celestial harvest claimed.

Going Barton one better was a fasting girl by the name of Eva Vliegen (1575–1637), who lived in Meurs, a small town on the Rhine river in Germany. Physician Guilhelmus Fabricius Hildanus (1560–1634), renowned as the 'Father of German Surgery', took up Vliegen's case. The patient told him that she relied on a single source of sustenance even more ethereal than Barton's own – the scent of flowers. Both cases met with healthy scepticism on the part of their respective investigators. Their scepticism turned out to be completely warranted: both Barton and Vliegen proved frauds. The discovery likely inspired Weyer to give his report on Barton's case the exposé-like title, 'On Alleged Fasting'.

Though the bogus nature of the diets observed by these fasting girls came to light, their cases did serve to stoke interest in fasting itself. Its mysteries attracted minds of greater and lesser scientific bents. Amateurs joined experts in an eagerness to see and measure the effects of diet on the human organism. The questions they were investigating did have a certain irresistibility. What was this mysterious process that could dispense with food as disparate as mutton, blancmange and wine? What explained the fact that some individuals could go months without food, whereas others grew ill after only a few hours? Such queries occupied inquiring minds – be they trained in emerging medical and health-related disciplines or wholly innocent of such learning – and drove them to creative experimentation.[22]

The Effects of Different Foods

Eating added weight to the human frame, whereas not eating removed it – this much had been established at least since Erasistratus. Yet another question lingered, begging to be answered: did different foods have different effects, beyond the adding and removal of weight? The eighteenth-century English physician William Stark (*c.* 1740–1770) sought to answer this question. Intrigued by Benjamin Franklin's claim to have lived successfully for a fortnight on nothing but bread and water, Stark changed his diet every few weeks and dutifully noted the results.

For the first two weeks Stark followed Franklin's example and lost 1.6 kilograms (3½ lb). He then sweetened the austere fare with sugar, the addition of which caused Stark to shed the same amount again. The weight loss came accompanied by other ill effects – abscesses on his gum, for one. Diarrhoea followed a switch to bread and olive oil as sole sustenance; the condition reversed only after Stark added water once again and abandoned olive oil for roast goose. The latter diet restored him to a state 'hearty and vigorous, both in mind and body'.[23] Stark carried on his adventures in gastronomy for six months, the menus growing more baroque all the while. Egg yolks and suet, figs and water, bread, fat and jelly – these were just some of the odd combinations he ate, possibly to his detriment; he eventually developed a fever that led to his death.

The sadness of Stark's death perhaps resulting from his experiment in restricted diets may have been compounded by his failure to arrive at any definite scientific discoveries in human digestion. The whole endeavour simply left him with a distaste for austere eating as inherently unpleasant. He noted shortly before his demise that Franklin and others must have embraced restricted diets as an escape from some experience even more unpleasant. He wrote that they must have been 'driven to' the 'temperance' that they practised 'as their last resource'.[24] What drove Stark to this conclusion was the belief, borne of his own experience, that 'nothing but the dread of former sufferings could have given them resolution to perseverance in so strict a course of abstinence'.[25] Not much by way of scientific knowledge had been advanced other than perhaps resounding proof that dieting was truly no fun.

Theories of Nutrition and Metabolism

More was put to the test in Santorio's and Stark's respective investigations than was discovered, especially in Stark's case. Yet it would not have been possible to glean more than a slight return in understanding, because those inquiries were subject to a particular limitation. This limitation owed to a reductive conception, dominant in the two experimentalists' time, that was materialist and mechanistic in its assumptions. This conception was that mechanical processes explain all phenomena, including human beings and animals, and that living beings existed as no more than mechanistic automata. This conception proved useful as far as it went. The trouble was that it went only part of the way. That is, it helped to establish the idea of nutrition and metabolism as exchanges of material and energy; yet it came up short in establishing the way in which the exchanges took place.

Further progress would have to await innovation on the materialist–mechanistic conception espoused by the likes of Santorio and Stark. Such innovation did arrive, courtesy of a blue-blooded French tax farmer by the name of Antoine-Laurent de Lavoisier (1743–1794).[26] Lavoisier elaborated a different theory to suit his keen inquisitiveness. It relied on quantitative measurement, and it abandoned mechanistic processes for chemical processes. Guided by this new approach, Lavoisier took up the challenge of explaining the invisible workings of human metabolism.

Lavoisier's investigations, commenced in the 1780s, began with breath. In partnership with the mathematician Pierre-Simon Laplace, the Frenchman devised a series of experiments on respiration. He placed guinea pigs in a chamber that was surrounded by layers of ice and had a funnel beneath it for catching any meltwater. This was Lavoisier's calorimeter – a device for measuring the heat of chemical reactions or physical changes – and it worked to show how much ice melted in a given time from the body heat of the guinea pig inside it. As the guinea pig abided in its ice-encrusted pen, Lavoisier measured the amount of oxygen the animal took in and the amount of carbon dioxide, or 'fixed air', it gave off. Following this, he took a lump of carbon that was the same size as a guinea pig, burned it and measured the amount of carbon dioxide it gave off. The amount of carbon dioxide given off by the burnt carbon turned out to be quite close to the amount of carbon dioxide from the guinea pig. The near equivalence led Lavoisier to conclude that his guinea pig subject produced the amount of carbon dioxide that it did in its exhalations by 'burning' that amount of carbon in its body.[27]

From this experiment Lavoisier formed a theory that respiration is slow combustion. He determined that the combustion took place in the lungs, and it supplied the rest of the body with heat.[28] This same combustion that happened in guinea pigs, Lavoisier reasoned, must happen in human beings, as well. To establish this commonality, Lavoisier found himself a human guinea pig. The lucky someone was chemist Armand Jean François Séguin (1767–1835). In the first experiment of its kind, Lavoisier fitted Séguin with a copper face mask, to which a rigid tube was attached. The assemblage collected its wearer's exhalations and conducted them to a mercury-filled eudiometer, a device for measuring changes in volumes of gas. Séguin wore it in three states: while his stomach was empty, after he had eaten and while he worked. In each of these states, Lavoisier would take Séguin's pulse, count his breathing rate and measure the amount of oxygen. Lavoisier found that the amount of oxygen measured was influenced by several factors, such as the amount of food that Séguin ate, the temperature of the room he happened to occupy and the amount of physical effort he devoted to any one task.[29] Séguin's patience did not end in vain; the experiment advanced understanding of the fundamental aspects of energy metabolism: work, heat and respiration.

Unfortunately, Lavoisier came to feel the heat of the French Revolution. He was led off to the guillotine in 1794 – all along the way begging a stay of two weeks so he might complete an experiment – and beheaded for alleged crimes stemming from his activities as a tax farmer. This came about a year after Communards shuttered the Académie des Sciences as a threat to the state. His execution was decried by the physiologist Charles Richet as the most criminal act of the Revolution. Lavoisier's friend Joseph-Louis Lagrange (1736–1813) expressed a similar sentiment when he solemnly observed, 'It took but a second to cut off his head; a hundred years will not suffice to produce one like it.'[30]

While nature took her century to generate a suitable replacement head, the intellectual fruits of the lost original managed to endure the same span of years. Begun in earnest was the science of measuring the amount of heat released or absorbed during a chemical reaction – a science which came to be known as calorimetry. Lavoisier located the reaction in the lungs, although he never managed to observe the reaction's exact process.[31] Other scientists would follow in his wake and doggedly explore the chemical and physical reactions and mechanisms of human digestion.

Mysteries of Metabolism

These explorations gained in urgency with the development of political and economic forces that made life increasingly difficult to sustain. England's Inclosure Act of 1773 was followed by starvation. The statute barred the English peasantry from land that it had previously hunted on and farmed in common. Around the same time on the European continent, food prices climbed upward because fewer hands were available to work the land. Hunger ensued. In response to the crisis, Lavoisier's spiritual heirs tackled the problem of feeding more people in the face of fewer resources. They imagined the key to a solution to lie in fathoming the mystery of human metabolism.

Chemists weren't alone in meeting the challenge of the moment. As they concerned themselves with nutrition and metabolism, physiologists were making inroads into the study of the digestive system. Rather than invisible chemical reactions, physiologists focused on the observable functions of the body – and their experiments could be accordingly gruesome. To mark the dissolution of flesh by gastric juices, American physician John Richardson Young (1782–1804) placed the legs of a living frog into a bullfrog's stomach. Young observed that the flesh on those legs remained intact. From this, he deduced that only dead flesh was subject to gastric dissolution.[32]

Similarly keen on understanding the action of gastric juices, the Italian physiologist Lazzaro Spallanzani (1729–1799) devised an experiment in which he stuffed small linen sacks with food. Once they were full, he cinched the end of each sack closed and attached a length of string to it. He then stuffed the secured sacks down the throats of animal subjects as various as fish, frogs, newts, snakes, birds, sheep, oxen, cats and dogs. Spallanzani periodically hoisted the sacks out of the stomachs of his animal subjects by the lengths of string. He did this to check the state of dissolution of the food within the sacks. As if to share in the misery he inflicted on his animal subjects, Spallanzani also swallowed sacks of food to note the effects of his own gastric juices.[33]

Other physiologists dispensed with animal subjects. They may have been guided in this decision by the availability of human subjects who lent themselves to inquiry. American physician Edward Stevens (1754–1834), for example, believed himself to have found the perfect subject – a man who swallowed stones for a living. Stevens persuaded the man to abandon stones for silver tubes. Stevens put food in these tubes, which he would fetch from the man's stool some 36 to 48 hours after their ingestion. Later, in the nineteenth century, fellow American physiologist William Beaumont (1785–1853) was even luckier to come upon a man named Alexis St. Martin. A voyager by vocation, St. Martin lived with a hole in his stomach that came as the result of a gun-shot.[34] Beaumont would peer into this ghastly hole to watch digestive processes at work.

Chossat's Theory of Digestion

Despite all the swallowing of food-filled tubes and peering into unhealed gunshot wounds, adequately detailed and systematic experiments on digestion only came about in the work of the nineteenth-century Swiss physiologist, physician and politician Charles Chossat (1796–1875). Chossat dealt a blow to Lavoisier's theories when in 1820 he conducted a series of gruesome experiments for his thesis at the Faculté de Médecine in Paris. Not content with Lavoisier's chemical theories of respiration, Chossat wanted to advance a theory he could support with visible proof. To this end, he set about revealing to the world the intricate flesh-and-blood functions of living organisms.[35]

If we know anything of human nutrition and metabolism, it is thanks to countless dogs, pigeons, frogs, snakes, apes, cats, rats and mice that were flayed, bisected, starved, suffo-cated, drugged and otherwise mutilated. Scientific inquiry's very nature breeds cruelty; only a cultivated disinterest and devotion to the betterment of the human condition set the scientist apart from the sadist. (English scientist Robert Hooke was so saddened by his experiment of cutting a dog's trachea that he vowed never again to repeat it.) Chossat was no exception in this respect. His experiments were shockingly cruel. One of his inquiries called for plunging dogs into cold water baths time and again until they perished, all for a better understanding of 'death by cooling'. Another saw dogs having their spines severed at several points, after which their temperature was monitored for their rate of cooling as they died.[36] Chossat found that when he ligatured the thoracic aorta, which supplies blood to the abdominal muscles, the lungs cooled faster than the abdomen.[37] Despite the horrific deeds involved, this second experiment rendered an important discovery – in fact, the very revelation Chossat had been hoping for. He demonstrated that it was not the lungs that supplied the body with its heat, as Lavoisier had claimed, but the stomach. The engine of the body's supply of heat, consequently, was digestion rather than respiration.

Following his discovery of digestion as the source of body heat in 1820, Chossat went on to do only a few more experiments on death by cooling; he preferred his physician's practice to the laboratory. His retirement from experimentation proved short-lived, however. Through the intervening years, his digestion theory nagged at him, eventually compelling him to return to the laboratory around 1840, this time to focus on starvation.

Chossat's Inquiry into Underfeeding and Starvation

Guiding Chossat's new inquiry were two questions: what did
an animal experience if it was deprived of food? And what
did it experience if it was given food in insufficient amounts?
He began by observing the feeding habits of various animals.
Turtle doves, for example, he observed to eat 10 per cent of
their weight in food; pigeons, a little over 7.5 per cent. Along
with the amounts of food that different animals ate, he also
recorded the frequency with which they did so. Some ate
several times a day, whereas others – reptiles, most notably
– went weeks without doing so.[38] Drawing on the insights
gained in his earlier investigations into digestion, Chossat
concluded that it was the animals with the highest body
temperatures that ate not only the most, but the most often.

From this conclusion, Chossat proceeded to the experiment proper. He collected guinea pigs, pigeons, rabbits, turtle
doves, frogs, snakes and tortoises: more than one hundred
animals in all, each locked away in an individual cage. Once
Chossat had thus secured all his animal subjects, he moved
to the next stage, which was that of denying them food.
As they starved, he observed their condition. His animal
subjects lost the most weight early in the experiment, a
reduction that Chossat attributed to their bowel movements.
Following this early precipitous drop, weight loss continued
at a steady rate until the animal died. Regardless of species,
every animal perished once it grew 40 per cent lighter than
its original weight. Mammals met this end after fifteen to
eighteen days. Reptiles, meanwhile, took well over a year
to arrive at this eventuality.

Whether it took a fortnight or a year, the path from the initial denial of food to death followed much the same progression in each of Chossat's animal subjects, regardless of species. The animal remained calm in the early stages. When it reached the midway point between its final meal and impending death, however, it grew agitated and continued in this state as long as its body temperature remained high. As death neared and the animal grew weak, its body temperature dropped. A stupor overtook the animal, and, as Chossat noted, it looked around as if in unbelief about its state.[39] Blank staring ceded to a seeming sleep; the animal closed its eyes, no longer able to stand. Any attempt to get to its feet caused it to tremble. Chossat's birds, for example, rested quietly on their bellies and wings. At some point, even this took too much effort. They then fell on their sides, their feet livid and balled, and died.[40] In an added twist of cruelty, no accompanying wasting of the brain appeared to afflict Chossat's birds. They looked as if they registered all that happened around them.

Chossat sometimes tried to revive moribund birds by warming them in an oven. The gentle heat brought them around. He offered them food, which they took, and it seemed to restart the mechanism of digestion. Yet the birds were usually too far gone by then. So advanced was their starvation, and so cold their bodies, that they died anyway. Necropsies that Chossat performed on the tiny, wasted bodies revealed that the birds' hearts had been most significantly affected by the starvation. The hearts had grown smaller, sacrificed to the energy needs of the nervous system, which Chossat observed to have remained unscathed. He further noted that the same effects took hold whether an animal was starved or underfed.[41] The sole difference was the time it took for the animal subject to die – longer from underfeeding and shorter from starvation.

The sacrifice of his many animal subjects ultimately redounded to the glory of the man who starved and underfed them. The investigations won Chossat wide praise, as well as the gold medal for Experimental Physiology from Paris' Royal Academy of Sciences in 1841. 'These experiments are believed to prove in the most satisfactory manner both the use and the destination of food, and to show that its object is essentially to maintain the animal temperature,' a reviewer for the *Edinburgh Medical and Surgical Journal* wrote in 1844.[42] 'It cannot escape observation, nevertheless, that to ascertain the utility of food scarcely required a series of experiments so elaborate,' the reviewer hastened to add. 'Any person of common observation knows that the great use of food is to supply the constant waste to which the system is incessantly exposed.'[43] Common observation may have made this tendency obvious, but it took the uncommon observation of Chossat to reveal the outcome of constant waste when it went unchecked by any such resupply.

A Growing Body of Knowledge about Human Nutrition

As Chossat was depriving the last of his birds and snakes of vital nutrients, Justus von Liebig (1803–1873) was just getting started on some animal subjects of his own. In the 1840s, the German chemist set his sights on human nutrition in the hope of preventing the famines of the past.[44] To that end, he conducted a series of experiments designed to discover the effects wrought by malnutrition. The experiments involved feeding animal subjects – dogs, in this instance – various diets, each of which was missing certain vital nutrients. Observation of the effects led Liebig to theorize that the nutrients needed by animals and human beings alike were three: protein, carbohydrates and fat.[45] Protein built and repaired tissue, whereas fats and carbohydrates served as fuel. The lack of any of the three in a diet brought on death.

Nothing short of revolutionary, Liebig's discoveries established the importance of certain classes of food, as well as the amount of oxygen needed to burn that food. Food, oxygen and various chemicals in the body: from the interaction of these arose life. This profound insight served to clinch Liebig's enduring influence on nutrition and nutritional chemistry.[46]

Scientists who followed in Liebig's footsteps added to the growing body of knowledge of human nutrition. The latter half of the nineteenth century saw them employ techniques developed by Lavoisier to pursue such avenues of inquiry as the physiology of digestion, the importance of certain nutrients and the speed at which the body converted certain nutrients to energy. They also sought to answer the question of what happened when people failed to get enough to eat. Accounts of starvation had heretofore largely concerned themselves with its corrosive social effects. 'A brother rose against his brother, a father had no pity for his son, mothers had no mercy for their daughters; one denied his neighbor a crumb of bread,' reads a thirteenth-century Russian chronicle of a famine in the Ukrainian city of Novograd. 'It was a bitter sight, indeed, to watch the crying children begging in vain for bread, and falling dead like flies.'[47] It is little wonder that records focused on such accounts of suffering by individuals and populations; perhaps this is in part why the biological implications of protracted hunger remained shrouded in mystery.

The shroud began to lift as the biological and psychological consequences of starvation grew in importance. One early investigator, Richard Baron Howard (1807–1848), studied the effects of semi-starvation on working-class men and women living in Manchester, England, in the 1830s. Howard was the physician at the Ardwick and Ancoats Dispensary, a factory in the industrial city, and so was able to study the workers at first hand. Howard noted in 1839 that they suffered 'languor, exhaustion, and general debility' when underfed – a state into which these workers often fell, owing to long bouts of unemployment and a consequent inability to buy food.[48] The debility presented as chills, poor balance and a 'weak and tremulous' voice.[49] The evil consequences didn't end there. Howard's starved workers also experienced mental slowness, bodies that had 'shrunk' and haggard faces whose features had 'collapsed'.[50] Finally – as was also true of Chossat's animal subjects – Howard's famished workers were 'startled by any sudden noise and hurried by the most trifling occurrences', such was the nervousness that beset them.[51]

Howard's study of Mancunian factory hands yielded important details on how starvation affected human beings, yet the most detailed accounts of human starvation would come from a study of workers of a different kind: polar explorers. The scientifically minded explorers dutifully recorded the effects of the famine they endured during their expeditions, which often met with extreme hardship. Such was the case with the Greely Arctic Expedition. In the summer of 1883, the expedition's leader, A. W. Greely, and his team came to the end of their expedition and awaited a steamship that never arrived. That ship was the *Proteus*, and it failed to reach the rendezvous point on Lady Franklin Bay, an Arctic waterway in Nunavut, Canada.[52]

Unable to get home or access fresh supplies, Greely and crew found themselves forced to winter in the frozen wastes. 'Our constant talk is about something to eat, and the different dishes we have enjoyed, or hope to enjoy on getting back to civilization,' an expedition member by the name of Lieutenant Lockwood would later recall. 'We are hungry all the time.'[53] Their rations nearly exhausted by October, the men grew irritated and distrustful. They accused each other of stealing food from the commissary house. 'We are all more or less unreasonable, and I only wonder that we are not all insane,' wrote another member of the crew. Scurvy soon set in, and one by one they began to die of starvation, several of them eking out a few additional weeks of life by eating rock tripe (a nutrient-rich lichen) and reindeer moss that returned with spring. Sooner or later, death came, and as it approached, the doomed, starving crew members ceased to feel pangs of hunger. Of the 25 members of the Greely Expedition, only seven survived to be rescued on 23 June 1884. One rescue party member described Greely as grimy and hollow-eyed, 'his hair . . . long and matted', and 'his feet and joints . . . swollen'.[54] As it happened, the party arrived just in the nick of time. Had they been delayed for even 48 hours, they would have found Greely dead.[55]

The story of the Greely Expedition and similar accounts of gruelling polar treks revealed much about the physical and psychological effects of starvation. Yet they also distorted the phenomenon a bit. Polar explorers starved under conditions rife with unique stressors, such as fear and exposure to the elements. These stressors served to aggravate the effects of starvation – and to speed them up, as well. Under conditions of famine, then, the effects of starvation alone couldn't be adequately isolated.

Willing Participants

Fortunately for science, the nineteenth century saw the ascent of a class of men and women who starved willingly, even happily, under normal conditions. They were the hunger artists, and they earned their bread (which they didn't eat) by fasting for the entertainment of others. (If we remember their existence today, it is because of Franz Kafka's 1922 story 'A Hunger Artist'.)

The most famous hunger artist of the time was Giovanni Succi (1853–1918). He likely served as the model for Kafka's protagonist and inspired modern-day fasters like David Blaine. Succi took to fasting while seeking a cure for unnamed ailments he had developed during his youthful wanderings in Africa. Believing himself possessed by a benign spirit that helped him live without food – a claim that often led to his confinement in mental institutions – he became an ardent devotee of the practice. From 1886, Succi travelled throughout Europe to show off his ability to fast for thirty days at a time. Onlookers marvelled at how placidly he could endure hunger.[56]

It was this quality that led Dr Francis Gano Benedict (1870–1957), director of the Carnegie Nutrition Laboratory, to consider Succi an ideal candidate for participation in what he hoped would be (and did become) the most exhaustive study of starvation theretofore completed. Succi's devotion to adding to scientific knowledge, however, wasn't nearly so ardent as his devotion to adding to his personal wealth. Aware of his star status, he demanded an unreasonably high payment for his participation. This forced Benedict to approach someone else in 1911. The person Benedict settled on was an eccentric Maltese lawyer and labour agitator named Agostino Levanzin (1872–1955).

Levanzin had an unconventional background. The son of a dockworker, and no stranger to all the privations and extremities of poverty, Levanzin dedicated himself from his early youth to the proletarian cause. When he was still a teenager, he published a newspaper called *A Friend to All*, which he intended to educate and enlighten its working-class readers. It failed, but by then Levanzin had decided to become a cleric. 'Matter of convictions and bigoted tyranny of the superiors', however, made him change his mind about taking holy orders.[57]

Levanzin turned to the professions, studying pharmacy and, after he found himself ill-suited to compounding drugs for querulous invalids, law. All the while he continued a host of side pursuits: starting – and later shuttering – newspapers dedicated to his sundry interests, writing novels, lecturing, founding societies, promoting women's rights and agitating for better conditions for the working classes. In service to this last cause Levanzin was even jailed for denouncing corruption in the dockyards in which his father had worked. A life thronging with commitments could exhaust a man. And Levanzin was indeed exhausted. Rather than easing off, however, he sought to boost his flagging energy by stuffing himself with obscene amounts of milk, eggs and meat. Yet the heavy diet only added to his exhaustion. In fact, as he later told Benedict, it dealt his nervous system 'a severe shock of neurasthenia'.[58] He had grown obese and pessimistic, and was unable to work.

Having exchanged exhaustion for total incapacity, Levanzin was desperate for a solution. 'It was then I discovered fasting,' he said. 'It was a flash of light that struck me vividly.'[59] His first fast lasted eight days with 'very great benefit'.[60] He then went on a 'conquest fast' for forty days with the intention of subduing the ills that plagued him. His wife, who sought to cure her severe dyspepsia and insomnia, joined him for the first 33 of those forty days. By the end of their fasts, both found that their ailments had vanished.

Levanzin ate heartily in the days preceding the fast for Benedict's study, despite having told Benedict he usually followed a spare vegetarian diet. But blaming the sea voyage to Boston for upsetting his usual eating routine, Levanzin gorged on salmon and pork and lamb chops. On one occasion prior to beginning the fast, he ordered large portions of macaroni, fried sweet potatoes and fried aubergine, along with two slices of French bread, two portions of butter, one portion of chocolate ice cream, a half-dozen macaroons and five glasses of water. His appetite was all the more impressive given that, only a few hours before, he had eaten broiled salmon, a number of pork chops, mashed potatoes, a portion of cucumbers and tomatoes, three rolls and a strawberry ice cream.[61]

Levanzin could hardly be blamed for his gluttony. The next day he entered Benedict's calorimeter room, which was to be his home for the next 31 days. And for those 31 days he would take nothing but water. He filled the time as best he could. When he wasn't in the calorimeter box, he worked on his autobiography, read and rested. Sometimes he went on a car ride with Benedict's laboratory assistants or stepped on to the roof for fresh air. He also underwent a battery of tests – blood, urine, respiration, finger-tapping, memory – as well as X-rays and measurements of his bodily proportions. He did baulk at certain tests. He wouldn't engage with the dynamometers used to test muscular strength, for example, claiming he was a 'professional gentleman' and therefore unaccustomed to muscular work.[62]

Levanzin showed himself an able faster, remaining remarkably healthy throughout the study. 'The blood as a whole is able to withstand the effects of complete abstinence from food for a period of at least 31 days without displaying any essentially pathological change,' Benedict concluded from observing his subject's state.[63] Indeed, the only pathological change shown by Levanzin during his 31-day fast was mental agitation. He even claimed to enjoy the fast because during it he came to believe that food 'impedes the body and mind and animal food is poison' (perhaps he was recalling the mounds of food he had eaten in the days before the fast).

He thus fasted in the faith that 'the poison of the food I have eaten will be eliminated, my body cleaned of its impurities, and my mind will be free and active.'[64] But this confidence in the healthfulness of his fast did waver at times. On the fast's seventh day, for example, he became 'mentally depressed'; 'extreme mental depression' appeared again for a brief period after the fast.[65]

Surprisingly, despite this change of mood, Levanzin was loath to break the fast when it came to an end. He appeared downcast as he took his first meal of orange and lemon juice, grape juice and honey. He felt it dangerous to break a fast before a true desire for food had returned, and even after 31 days without food, he still wasn't hungry. (Indeed, he claimed to have experienced few to no hunger pangs during his fast.) And perhaps he was right: the days following the termination of his fast, during which he consumed small amounts of food, saw him afflicted with cramps, vomiting, diarrhoea, colic, feelings of lassitude and depression, weakness, insomnia and, finally, disappointment. His disappointment, however, had nothing to do with his fast itself but with its reception. 'He was plainly disappointed', Benedict wrote, 'because the world had not given him the recognition due him for the sacrifice he had made for the benefit of mankind.'[66]

Although Levanzin himself might not have received the attention he thought he deserved, the Carnegie Nutrition Study would come to be recognized as one of the most important and exhaustive studies on human starvation. And although the study would later be criticized for not giving adequate time to pre-experiment training, it yielded many noteworthy findings, the most important of which was that, under the right conditions, a human could fast for long periods with little lasting physical or mental consequence.[67]

The Carnegie study would inspire other important experiments on fasting and starvation. In 1916, College of the City of New York researcher Howard Marsh and his wife May reduced their food consumption over three weeks, eating nothing during the second week of the experiment to see whether fasting affected the sexes differently. Marsh observed that May's memory improved, whereas his own did not.[68] Twelve years later, the wife of University of Michigan scientist John Arthur Glaze (1887–1973), identified only as 'A', and a 35-year-old man, identified only as 'C', who had previously fasted off and on for some three hundred days, subjected themselves to an experiment on the effects of fasting on the psyche and one's sense of smell. Glaze found that the latter became markedly heightened.[69]

The few studies into starvation revealed a lot about the phenomenon's psychological and physiological effects. And they delivered the added benefit of revealing much about human nutrition. Indeed, the science of the second depended on the science of the first. American physiologist and nutritionist Graham Lusk (1866–1932) insisted as much: 'Nutrition may be defined as the sum of the processes concerned in the growth, maintenance, and repair of the living body as a whole or of its constituent organs,' he wrote in his 1906 book *The Elements of the Science of Nutrition*. 'An intelligent basis for the understanding of these processes is best acquired by a study of the organism when it is living at the expense of materials stored within itself, as it does in starvation.'[70]

Yet these experiments on hunger artists and the understanding spouses of scientists still had a way to go. Although scientists finally found subjects who would starve willingly, there lingered several questions about experimental design. Could knowledge learned from a single subject, or even a handful of subjects, be generalized to humankind as a whole? Where were the controls? How could one account for the physiological and psychological idiosyncrasies of the subjects involved? Each question pointed out real shortcomings of the experiments as they had been conducted. What was needed was a large study that enlisted dozens of subjects. Finding two or three consenting subjects was difficult enough, however; finding scores of them, exponentially more so.

The Turnip Winter, 1916–17

Where recruitment for starvation studies failed, history supplied the inspiration. The studies of Dr Francis Gano Benedict and his contemporaries happened to coincide with the events of the First World War. The grinding conflict brought famine, among other woes. In Germany alone, where poor weather and a shortage of fertilizers led to crop failures, millions of men and women suddenly found themselves gripped with hunger. The crisis lasted from 1916 to 1917. The coldest months of that stretch were dubbed 'the turnip winter', so named for the vegetable that replaced the usual cereal grains and potatoes.

Shocked by the humanitarian disaster unfolding in Europe, Benedict set out to discover ways to remedy it. He once again turned his attention to studying the effects of semi-starvation. Benedict made it his goal, as he wrote, to 'instill into the world at large a belief that a pronounced lowering of rations is not necessarily accompanied by a complete disintegration of the organism'.[71] In other words, Benedict wanted to prove that people didn't need to eat as much as they thought they did; that, indeed, their bodies could adapt to a restricted diet, thus allowing for greater use of what rations were available.

In 1917 Benedict decided to test his theory. He recruited 24 male college students and placed them on a restricted diet, which, he intended, would make them lose 10 per cent of their total weight over a series of months. Benedict's subjects ate largely the same foods as their fellow students, only in smaller quantities.[72] After a few weeks they showed clear signs of semi-starvation: irritability, sensitivity to cold, weakness and lack of interest in sex. Otherwise, they seemed to do fine on reduced rations.

For all the altruism that motivated Benedict, his latest experiment suffered flaws. For one, he allowed his subjects to go home for the Thanksgiving and Christmas holidays, trusting that they would continue to observe their diet. (They disappointed him in this regard; they arrived back to campus heavier than they left.) For another, Benedict never thought to measure his subjects' consumption of fats and carbohydrates. Despite its flaws, the experiment saw many of the participants noticeably thinner by its end.[73] More importantly, it helped to lay the groundwork for studies to follow.

The wavering resolve of Benedict's male starvation study subjects served as a stark reminder of how difficult it is to get individuals to endure hunger willingly. All the more difficult, then, was to find individuals willing to endure hunger to the point of death.

The Jewish Hospital Czyste

History would intervene a few decades later with a tragic boon in the form of unwilling subjects whose starvation endured to its fatal end. Physicians from the medical and pediatrics departments of the Jewish Hospital Czyste in Warsaw, Poland, devised, from February to July 1942, a series of investigations into the effects of starvation. By undertaking the study, the investigators were making a virtue of necessity: patients being treated in the medical care facility were being starved by the Nazi German occupiers of Poland, as were the physicians themselves. For some time prior to the study, these physicians and patients, like all the occupants of the Warsaw ghetto, received meagre rations of dark bread, rye flour, buckwheat cereal, potatoes, and miserly amounts of butter, lard, oil and sugar. The diet was almost devoid of protein and fat, two of the elements that Liebig had declared, one hundred years before, to be essential to life. The rations offered each person only 800 calories, 3 grams of fat and 20 to 30 grams of vegetable protein (the average adult needs about 60 grams a day).

The physicians at the Jewish Hospital Czyste meticulously recorded the effects of this meagre fare, marking progress of edema (swelling caused by fluid in the body's tissues), changes in temperature, changes in pulse rate and changes in blood pressure and volume. They also observed how their patients lay in bed, moved around and reacted to stimuli.[74] Many of their studies survived only in fragments; others went uncompleted as the physicians themselves were sent to death camps. The surviving parts nonetheless offer a sombre glimpse into the progress of starvation.

The physicians remarked that they watched helplessly as their patients' starvation progressed in cruel stages. First, as had been noted almost a century earlier in Chossat's starving pigeons, surplus fat disappeared. 'This stage was reminiscent of the time before the war when people went to Marienbad, Karlsbad, or Vichy for a reducing cure and came back looking younger and feeling better,' they noted.[75] This was followed by a stage 'in which the patients looked old and withered', and then finally by 'hunger cachexia' – a profound wasting of muscle and fat – in the terminal stage.[76] And all the while there appeared painful and maddening symptoms: skin so dry that when it was rubbed by a fingernail it raised a large weal; a tongue turned a dirty brown and a body sheathed in a 'luxuriant fuzz' of fine hair; slack muscles; a persistent chill deep within; teeth riddled with caries; a mask-like expression with eyes clouded by cataracts.[77] The patients' mouths were parched with constant thirst while fluids pooled in their extremities. The fluids swelled their feet and hands to grotesque sizes, an effect that served to conceal the markers of emaciation. And all the while they 'vanished like a melting wax candle', the physicians noted.[78]

The physicians of the Jewish Hospital did this work knowing that they too would very likely die – of hunger, in the camps or in some other unspeakable way. Their investigations into starvation were an act of defiance, a way of doing good amid great evil. 'And you by your work could give the henchman the answer "Non omnis moriar," "I shall not wholly die,"' Dr Milejkowski, the head physician, wrote in a note preceding the study.[79] And these words proved prophetic. In 1979 physician Myron Winick noted that the parts of the study that survived have proven to 'constitute probably the best clinical description of the effects of severe semistarvation published in the medical literature to that date and perhaps even to the present'.[80]

Minnesota Starvation Experiment

Across the Atlantic, American physiologist Ancel Keys (1904–2004) had taken note of the horrific situation once again gripping Europe. Today Keys is best known for developing K-rations (used by the u.s. military during the Second World War) and popularizing the Mediterranean diet. But in November 1944, Keys concerned himself with developing a way to feed the starving masses of Europe. With this aim in mind, he welcomed to the University of Minnesota's Laboratory of Hygiene 36 conscientious objectors who had responded to the call of his recruiting pamphlet. The pamphlet was entitled 'Will You Starve That They Be Better Fed?', and these college-aged men who answered yes would participate in one of the most thorough studies on the effects of starvation in willing volunteers.

The Minnesota Starvation Experiment, as it came to be called, lasted a little over a year. It started with a three-month control period, in which the volunteers were given a daily allotment of 3,492 calories consisting of 124 grams of fat,

112 of protein and 482 of carbohydrates. They were then placed on a six-month semi-starvation diet consisting of bran bread, potatoes, cereals, turnips and cabbage, and the occasional smattering of meat, butter and sugar. With most of the 1,570 calories coming from carbohydrates, this diet was only slightly more generous than that eaten by the Jews of the Warsaw ghetto, and was generally on par with other famine diets. (The diet was intended to make the men lose 24 per cent of their body weight – significantly more than the 10 per cent Benedict had expected from his collegiate volunteers.) These rations were divided into two meals a day, at 8:30 a.m. and 5:00 p.m. The study participants were encouraged to do as they wished between the two meals, so long as they didn't snack or otherwise sneak food.

The men experienced the usual effects of starvation. Keys's account of the experiment is replete with photographs of young men grown cadaverous, the stress of food deprivation marring their faces. But what is most interesting to the lay reader are Keys's extensive notes on the psychological effects of starvation. All the volunteers were, in one way or another, idealistic, intellectually curious, ambitious men. Many came from close-knit Mennonite and Quaker communities. One wanted to go into the ministry; another aimed to become a rural cooperative farmer. Yet months of starvation turned them strangely obsessive. Some took to collecting menus and cookbooks, reading the descriptions of dishes and recipes as though they were highbrow literature.[81] Others collected cooking paraphernalia: coffee pots, hot plates, kitchen utensils.[82] As the weeks passed, their behaviour became yet more bizarre. Many grew suspicious and mean. 'We are no longer

polite,' said one participant.[83] One man repeatedly dreamt
of eating senile and insane people, savouring their flesh 'like
good pie or rare steak'.[84] Another hacked off three fingers
from his left hand.[85] Yet another confessed 'impelling desires
to smash or break things'.[86] All looked with desperation to
the refeeding period.

Yet refeeding would present its own problems. Unlike
the semi-starvation diet, not everyone received the same
amount of food. The men were split into groups, one of
which received 400 extra calories, another 800. The luckiest
groups received a relatively generous 1,200 and 1,600
additional calories.[87] There were other differences as well.
Some of the men received additional vitamin supplements;
others received more protein. But regardless of amount, the
extra food worked its effect: steadily the men gained weight,
with those who received the most food naturally gaining the
fastest. Apathy disappeared, replaced by a restive querulous-
ness. Still, fatigue, depression, low sex drive and a constant
gnawing hunger all remained.

Curiously, with the restorative diet the study participants
added weight mainly as fat. Some were never again as fit as
they had been before the experiment, their muscle replaced
by a 'soft roundness'.[88] What's more, the groups receiving
extra protein and vitamins recovered their strength no faster
than those who received no such supplementation.[89] Only
extra calories sped recovery. The men fed the most food
regained their physical and psychological health the fastest.[90]

Upon being released from the programme the men
ate whatever they wished, and in whatever amounts they
wished, often eating more than their shrunken stomachs

could handle. They inhaled snacks between large meals.[91] They drank milk in 'remarkable quantities'.[92] One subject had to limit his exposure to food, for he 'could not find a point of satiation even when he was "full to the gills"'.[93] And when they ate, they had little regard for manners, wolfishly gobbling and licking and gulping their food. 'This gluttony resulted in a high incidence of headaches, gastrointestinal distress, and unusual sleepiness,' noted Keys.[94] Many of the men vomited after eating; one required 'aspiration and hospitalization for several days'; and another, having eaten upwards of 10,000 calories a day, almost taxed his weakened heart to failure.[95] Only after 33 weeks in recovery did the study participants resume more-or-less normal eating habits.

The volunteers of the Minnesota Experiment suffered harrowing effects from their months-long semi-starvation diet. But they also experienced a few curiously beneficial effects: they had fewer cavities and their cholesterol decreased. Since the volunteers were already essentially healthy, however, these changes were slight.

Health Benefits of a Limited Diet

In his 1950 write-up of the Minnesota Starvation Experiment, *The Biology of Human Starvation*, Ancel Keys noted the surprising beneficial effects of a limited diet in less healthy subjects. Towards the end of the First World War, there was a marked decrease in cancer rates in Germany. For people between sixty and seventy years old, the cancer rates were 10 to 12 per cent higher in 1913 than in 1905.[96] But from 1915 to 1918, when food restrictions were put into place, the cancer mortality rate was low in all age groups, and only resumed its upward trend after the armistice.[97] Similar declines appeared during the Second World War. In Greece, cancer mortality decreased steadily after famine conditions appeared. A total of 990 people had died from cancer in 1940. In 1943, that number had decreased to 820.[98] All other major causes of death continued, meanwhile, to rise sharply.

These findings were intriguing. But even more intriguing were the data on diabetes and heart disease. Even during the first year of the Second World War there was a marked improvement in diabetes in patients living in Dresden and Würzburg.[99] In Belgium, from 1939 to 1942, total new cases of diabetes were reduced by half, especially among women.[100] Indeed, in the years preceding the war 68.5 per cent of diabetics were female; three years into the war this number had been reduced to 55 per cent.[101] Rates of heart disease also showed improvement. During the siege of Leningrad in 1941–2 researchers noted that there was no significant change in hospital admissions for cardiovascular services and hypertension did not seem to be much changed, yet there was a marked decrease in coronary disease and heart attacks.[102]

Keys at first thought the low-fat nature of semi-starvation diets accounted for such reversals in ill health. But then he recalled that, when starving, the body consumes its own fat. He thus concluded these changes in health were likely due to a reduction in total calories. A fasting diet, if not taken to extremes, could vastly improve health.

This hunch of his would inspire numerous post-war studies into human nutrition and metabolism. As abundance replaced scarcity the emphasis would shift from ameliorating the effects of starvation to coping with the illnesses caused by overfeeding. For as the world recovered from the wreckage wrought by decades of social and economic upheaval, it would be too much food that would devastate the health and well-being of developed nations – a situation we are still living with today.

Fasting, meanwhile, would experience an interesting rehabilitation, going from a threat to public health to a means of securing it. This was old news, however, to those familiar with the practice. As we will see in the next chapter, for centuries people have used fasting as a means to cure ailments.

3

THE PHYSICIAN WITHIN: FASTING FOR HEALTH

'A little starvation can really do more for the average
sick man than can the best medicines and the
best doctors.'
– Mark Twain, 'My Debut as a Literary Person' (1903)[1]

As the twentieth century gave way to the twenty-first, the fruits of the starvation studies conducted in the earlier century attracted attention. These studies had been carried out against a backdrop of human suffering brought on by war; yet in times of relative peace the topic attracted people who, having learned of the preceding studies' results, showed themselves willing to endure, at least for some reasonable amount of time, the pangs of prolonged hunger in the hopes of improving some state or condition. In this chapter we'll explore the health benefits of fasting, along with the history of how we came to use those benefits to enhance our health and well-being.

One such person was the English writer Jeanette Winterson (b. 1959). During her fast as an inmate of southern Germany's Buchinger Wilhelmi fasting clinic in 2017, she told of waking cold and distraught one morning. So powerful were these feelings that she had begun to cry in her sleep. 'It is as though I am not just metabolizing worn-out cells and tissues but memory layers too,' she wrote at the time in her journal.[2] This astonishing biochemical feat came from Winterson's having endured two days at the clinic. Yet a morning cry wasn't to be her third day's only surprise. A glance in a mirror revealed that her skin had grown blotchy since her arrival, and her tongue somehow furred. Worse, she would have killed for a glass of wine.

Unhappily for Winterson, vegetable broth and warm water would have to do, as the clinic permitted no tippling. These she sipped throughout her eight-day supervised fast. And when they failed to fend off thoughts of food, she resorted to taking long walks or doing aerobics. Often, however, she would simply gaze at the waters of Lake Constance and fall into a reverie, stillness recommending itself over activity as the best way of coping.

Coping became easier after that fraught third day. 'Hunger is gone,' she noted on the fourth: 'true energy returns, and with it, optimism and a sense of humour.'[3] Recovered energy, optimism and humour buoyed her through the rest of her stay. In fact, the experience made her a convert. 'Short of giving up my entire life . . . and going zen on a mountain top somewhere, or nibbling Quorn and drinking water,' she wrote, 'fasting seemed the easiest option.'[4] Winterson now regularly exercises that option, fasting some four times yearly to keep her cholesterol and cortisol levels in check.

Benefits of Fasting

The media is rife with tales of the impressive health benefits of a good fast. A Thai fasting clinic left journalist Ian Belcher some 18 kilograms (40 lb) lighter after 170 foodless hours and fourteen enemas. He was possessed of 'an indecent amount of energy and . . . unnaturally bright eyes'.[5] And *New Yorker* writer Judith Thurman found herself 'in excellent spirits, squeaky-clean inside and out, with bright eyes, a flat stomach, and skin like a rose petal' upon ending her stay at a fasting clinic in California.[6]

Journalists on assignment aren't alone in their realization of the practice's benefits. News articles on fasting report how a 36-year-old marketing executive fasted 'six days in the month' to reach her target weight. Confining her day's eating to an eight-hour window, a 47-year-old composer realized increased energy and creativity. And eating restricted to a certain few hours – otherwise known as intermittent fasting – may have even cured a 46-year-old artist of her autoimmune disorder, if her testimony is to be believed. At the very least, we may take her at her word when she claimed that fasting 'has made a massive difference in my life'.[7] Countless similar testimonies are but a Google search away. And these anecdotal testimonies are buttressed by the numerous studies that have confirmed fasting's many health benefits.

Let's start with improved bloodwork. Studies showed that fasted animals with diabetes were cured of it, and fasted animals without diabetes showed increased insulin sensitivity and improved glucose tolerance. They also experienced drops in cholesterol and triglycerides, as well as lower blood pressure and resting heart rates.[8]

Fasting also promoted repair and rejuvenation. Injuries to spinal cords and brains were quicker to heal, and cardio-vascular functioning improved. Fasting also repaired damage to DNA, and contributed to the health of mitochondria, the powerhouses of our body's cells. Such improvements led fasted animals to live longer than their unfasted cage mates. And that increased longevity saw them more active and mentally alert as well.[9]

Researchers believe that such wonders owe to an increase in the sensitivity of insulin receptor signalling. In fasting animals, insulin more readily stimulates glucose uptake by muscle and liver cells, which use it as fuel. (The more readily glucose is taken up by these cells in your body, the less likely you are to develop metabolic disorders.) The better health brought by fasting is also likely related to autophagy, a metabolic process in which the body recycles parts of its own dead and worn-out cells, as well as to a boost in the population and diversity of beneficial bacteria in a fasting gut. These bacteria, which number in the trillions, in turn help to keep us healthy and trim.[10]

Most studies have been conducted on animals because human fasting studies suffer from high drop-out rates. The few human studies that do exist support the findings in animal studies. Just some of the observed benefits include reduced insulin resistance, resting heart rates and levels of such contributors to heart disease as glucose, insulin and homocysteine.[11]

These same benefits were seen in groups who, for religious reasons, regularly fast. Muslims observing *sawm* (a month-long period of Ramadan fasting) shed weight and lowered their cholesterol and blood glucose levels.[12] Mormons who follow fasting prescriptions likewise lowered their weight and blood glucose. And among their numbers appeared fewer cases of diabetes. Finally, the faith-based lifestyle of Seventh-Day Adventists, which includes a plant-based diet and daily fasting from late afternoon to morning, delivers blessings this side of paradise in the form of an additional 7.3 years of life on average.[13]

Such health benefits are impressive. It's strange to think, then, that we've only recently started to study the beneficial effects of fasting in any kind of systematic way. Yet in some cultures fasting has long been an important treatment for disease. This is especially true in India, where, as we shall see, physicians have long known that fasting is the cure for what ails you.

Ayurveda

Translated as 'the knowledge or science for longevity', Ayurveda represents one of history's first systematic, empirical approaches to medicine. Its roots lie in the Vedas, India's earliest literary record. This record, originally transmitted orally sometime between 1500 BCE and 800 BCE, came to be grouped into four major texts: the *Rigveda*, the *Samaveda*, the *Yajurveda* and the *Atharvaveda*. The *Atharvaveda* would in turn inform the golden age of Indian medicine, which ran from 800 BCE to 1000 CE. The *Atharvaveda* was a central influence on two thinkers: Caraka (*c.* second century CE), physician and author of the *Caraka-samhita*, and Sushruta (*c.* 800 BCE–700 BCE), surgeon and author of the *Sushruta Samhita* (*samhita* simply means 'a collection'). Though many other authorities would contribute to shaping Ayurvedic thought, the dominant influence of Caraka and Sushruta would persist undiminished through the centuries.

Their dominance rests on the fact that we find distilled in their respective works the fundamental ideas behind Ayurveda. This system holds that the universe's five constituent elements, or *pancha mahābhūtas* – air (*vayu*), earth (*prithvi*), ether (*akasha*), fire (*agni*) and water (*aap*) – combine to form every existing thing, be it organic or inorganic. The elements as they combine to form a human individual transmute into three semi-fluid substances known as *doshas* or humours. They are bile or choler (*pitta*), phlegm (*kapha*) and wind (*vāta*). Our sense of health and well-being depends on their remaining in a state of equilibrium. The same goes for our bodily tissues (*dhātu*) and waste (*mala*). 'When not in balance, the body tissues, the waste products, and the humours can destroy the body,' warns the *Sushruta Samhita*.[14] 'When balanced, they are known to promote happiness, strength, and growth.'[15] A ready and reliable way of restoring balance, as you may have already guessed, is fasting.

The Hindu scriptures have long considered fasting the supreme medicine for ridding the body of toxins. 'Whosoever fasts is blessed in every way,/ He draws the benefits of all the great medicines,/ All his diseases are cured and he becomes strong and virile,' reads a passage of the *Mahābhārata*, one of two Sanskrit epics of ancient India.[16]

The Hindu saint Dadhichi was said to have made his bones so strong by fasting that the king of gods, Indra, used them to fight demons.

Fasting's virtue for restoring balance and imparting strength rests on the Ayurvedic conception of digestion, in which the stomach works as something of an oven, cooking the food that enters it into a pulpy juice. The juice becomes blood. From blood issues flesh, and from flesh, fat. Some fat hardens to bone, which produces the marrow that in men becomes semen. Each stage of the transformation also produces humours, as well as waste and an oleaginous, fortifying energy known as *ojas*.[17]

Ojas, humours, waste and pulpy juice alike move about the body through a network of tubes. Should the network become clogged, the effect is akin to closing a fireplace's flue. The belly's digestive flame is dampened, which causes the entire apparatus to back up and slow down. (Imagine a shutdown of a major highway interchange during rush hour and you'll get the picture.) Enter fasting to the rescue. It empties the belly so that its fire may reignite to dry the accumulated fluids, and this quickly gets things moving again.

Care must be taken, however, because a fast's safety and effectiveness depend on your humoral profile. If it is one dominated by *kapha* (phlegm), then you can fast away; the practice will serve to lighten your otherwise 'heavy' nature.[18] If, on the other hand, yours is a constitution dominated by *pitta* (bile), you ought to fast with caution and mindfulness. The same holds for *vāta* (wind)-dominant individuals, pregnant women and the very old and young. Regardless of your age, condition or particular humoral mix, you must never prolong your fast. Doing so exhausts your body, thereby leaving it prone to new imbalances.

Ayurvedic authorities further recommend that you confine your fasts to the cool, moist months of spring. And during your time of fasting you should avoid sex and naps. You'll know your fast is going well by the delightful energy suffusing you and the feeling of lightness and purity in your heart, throat and mouth. You'll also belch lustily, sweat profusely and thrill with a keen appetite as your digestive fires reignite.[19] (If it is going poorly, you'll simply feel like crap.)

Similar prescriptions guided writer Jessica Berger Gross during her stay at the Ayurvedic Institute in Albuquerque, New Mexico. In *enLIGHTened: How I Lost 40 Pounds with a Yoga Mat, Fresh Pineapples, and a Beagle Pointer* (2012), she recalls how she had initially wished to go on a water-only fast. The institute's staff counselled against this, however, warning that it 'could shock and deplete the system rather than strengthen it'.[20] The fasting programme they crafted for her consisted of juices, potassium broth and grains, the last intended to rid her of toxins (*āma*) in a process called *kshut nigraha*, or holding and controlling one's hunger. 'At first, the juice fast sucked,' she admitted.[21] She did have cause to complain, though, bedevilled as she was early on by 'fatigue, chills, short-lived but piercing headaches, sensitivity to noise, people, and almost all outside stimulation'.[22] Three days and a few enemas later, she found she 'wasn't all that hungry'.[23] She claimed, rather, to have drawn nourishment from contact with fellow fasters at the institute, and this alone was enough to satisfy her.

Struggling with weight and food issues, Gross undertook her fast to avoid more serious health problems down the road. As it turned out, she acted in the very spirit of Ayurveda. Unlike more modern approaches, Ayurvedic medicine treats the patient, not the disease. The *Sushruta Samhita* characterizes the human body as 'the means of attaining virtue, wealth, pleasures, and liberation'.[24] For this very reason 'a man should be aware of the effects of his actions'.[25] Actions taken to promote his health and wellness thus have the effect of 'protect[ing] his body from diseases'.[26] Such wisdom has guided therapeutic fasting for centuries, helping Ayurveda to become the oldest continuously practised system of medicine. Indeed, some 80 per cent of Indians living today observe its regimens and prescriptions.[27]

Classical Antiquity

Western classical antiquity saw the development of preventive medicine strikingly reminiscent of Ayurveda. But unlike Ayurveda, this approach would not survive into the present – at least in the mainstream.

Views on fasting, as well as medicine generally, began to change around the fifth century BCE, when a more rational system of thought replaced a superstitious view of life and the universe. It was this new rationality that led the Greek physician Hippocrates to derive his treatments from observation and evidence rather than lore and tradition. One such treatment was fasting, its utility owing to the fact that for Hippocrates diet (*diaita*) presented the surest way to health. 'Let food be thy medicine, and medicine thy food' would become one of his most famous, albeit apocryphal, maxims. In the classical approach to weight loss, in both eating and fasting, discretion and moderation were key.

For classical physicians a proper diet was key to keeping open the conduits of the body's various humoral fluids. Like the physicians of India, from whom they likely received the idea, Greek physicians viewed the human body as a system akin to our modern water and sewerage systems, with inter-connected tubes conveying fluids and receptacles storing them. In one end arrived food, from which was distilled (you guessed it!) humours, which numbered four: blood; phlegm; yellow bile, or choler; and black bile, or melancholy. Waste exited the other end. Of course, this process presumed that the system operated smoothly. Humours determined an indi-vidual's temperament and state of health. Should a humour become blocked or pool in the wrong spot, an imbalance ensued, leaving the person affected feeling out of sorts or, worse, unwell.

The wise physician in his discretion sought the least injurious cure possible, so that he might live up to that other, albeit also likely apocryphal, Hippocratic maxim, 'Do no harm.'[28] Dietary adjustments therefore recommended them-selves as a treatment of first resort. Hippocrates counselled his patients to stay away from certain foods believed to cause an excess of this or that humour – beef and soft cheeses in cases of too much black bile, for example, or unripe apples in cases of too much phlegm. The physician urged few patients to forgo all food completely.

Any fasts that may have been called for tended to be brief. Hippocrates himself recommended that a patient first be put on a bland-food diet, which consisted solely of a thin barley gruel called *ptisane*.[29] If this didn't work, he next prescribed a water fast, albeit only if the patient was of a very old or very young age. Greek physician Galen (129–216 CE) likewise prescribed brief fasts for treating illness, and the Greek Stoic writer Plutarch (*c.* 46–120 CE), who lived in the days of the Roman Empire, allegedly counselled his audience, 'Instead of taking medicine, rather fast a day.'[30] He was likely echoing medical theories of the time. Patients were commonly made to fast for two days before they were given any further treatment.

The proviso that fasts be short didn't owe to any desire on the Greeks' part to get back to eating as quickly as possible (though you could hardly fault them if that had been the case). Rather, medical knowledge of their time held that brief fasts aided the body's natural healing powers, whereas extended fasts possibly hindered them. To their credit, ancient Greek physicians understood that individuals responded to fasts, well, individually. Some patients took to them, others didn't. Unpredictability of patient response meant it was wise to err on the side of caution, diagnostically speaking. Hippocrates, for example, feared that patients accustomed to three square meals a day might suffer dizziness, depression and 'listlessness', as well as 'hollowness of the eyes', hot urine, hanging bowels, weakness, lightheadedness and tremulousness, were they to fast.[31] (He may have seized here on the symptoms of hypoglycemia, known popularly as a 'sugar crash'.)

Those who fasted despite the dangers were regarded as bold. Those who fasted for long periods of time despite the dangers were regarded as insane. Heraclitus of Ephesus (*c.* 540–480 BCE), the pre-Socratic philosopher most known for observing that you cannot step in the same river twice, fled to the mountains, where he subsisted on grass and herbs. Onlookers labelled him as crazy. In fact, their snap judgement seemed to have been prescient because he also came down with edema, a swelling of tissues that suggested his humours had ceased to circulate.[32]

Heraclitus' alpine asceticism bred ill consequences because it violated the chief health and wellness ethic of his time: the exercise of restraint and understanding. Ancient Greek physicians laboured under the obligation to work with the body's mechanisms of recovery and self-repair, rather than against them – an obligation placed on them by none other than Hippocrates himself, who supposedly said that 'natural forces within us are the true healers of disease.' Fasting responded to the fact that most illness tends to curb the sufferer's appetite, so it was the treatment that was best suited to the sufferer's state. It thus presented a noninvasive and harmonious treatment. And though its virtues continued to be recognized well beyond the early Hellenic period into late imperial Rome, at some point they were forgotten. We turn now to discovering why this happened.

The short answer to the question of therapeutic fasting's lapse into oblivion is Christianity – or the rise of Christendom, to be exact. Yet it didn't sweep away existing medical knowledge so much as shape it to its own concerns, which were decidedly otherworldly. The fasting advice of pre-Christian ancients mingled with calls for mortifying the flesh as a way of currying favour with God and avoiding His punishment, the soul's health mattering more than the body's. Christian monks known as 'grazers', for example, lived on wild herbs alone – and they didn't grow healthier for it. Fasting regimes thus lost some of their secular character, as fasters adapted them to the aim of making themselves holy. You could say that, in a sense, the early Christian world returned fasting to its pre-classical status as a propitiatory act.[33]

We must look to the medieval Islamic world for survivals of therapeutic fasting in their classical secular character. Within its sphere flourished Arab scholars who did history the great service of recovering and translating works of the ancient Greek medical authorities. Their efforts also produced contributors of their own, among them the eleventh-century Muslim philosopher and physician Avicenna (Ibn Sīnā, 980–1037) and Moses Maimonides (1135–1204), a Jewish scholar who lived in Muslim Spain. They kept alive the empirical approach to medicine for later retrieval by the European scholars of the Renaissance, on whose minds the strict doctrines of Western Christianity had loosened a bit. These scholars translated the Arabic translations of the original Greek into Latin, the manuscripts of which they then had printed. Thanks to printing, the works perhaps found a wider audience than ever. And from them many readers drew inspiration to follow the examples set by Avicenna, Maimonides and others by developing their own secular theories of health and medicine.

Alvise (Luigi) Cornaro

The wealthy sixteenth-century Venetian architect and humanist Alvise (Luigi) Cornaro (1484–1566) was one such early advocate of a return to the classical approach to health and well-being. At first, he seemed an unlikely candidate. Until his fortieth birthday, Cornaro led a prosperous and dissolute life. Having made his fortune by designing hydraulics for wetlands reclamation – a real boon for a city like Venice – he ate, drank and fornicated to excess. His physicians naturally warned him off such a lifestyle, urging moderation. 'Impatient of such restraint', as he characterized himself, Cornaro spurned their warning. 'I could not put up with it,' he wrote of his younger self, 'and therefore eat freely of every thing I liked best.'[34]

But his excesses eventually caught up with him. By middle age his body was wracked with pain so severe that he wanted to die. He wrote of the 'different kinds of disorders' plaguing him. They included 'pains in my stomach, and often stitches, and spices of gout'.[35] Added to these were 'an almost continual slow fever, a stomach generally out of order, and a perpetual thirst'.[36]

Cornaro's condition had grown so acute that his physician shelved moderation, a remedy no longer adequate to the emergency, and instead commanded his patient to fast from all food liquid and solid. To choose to do otherwise was to choose death. A now-compliant Cornaro carried out the command faithfully and soon recovered – more than recovered, in fact. The radiant health restored to him by his fast prompted Cornaro to develop his own strict diet, which rested on the prescriptions of the classical authority Galen. To this end he resolved 'not to take of any thing, but as much as my stomach can easily digest, and to use those things only, which agree with me'.[37] The restrictions in practice amounted to a daily intake of a mere 340 grams (12 oz) of food chased by 414 millilitres (14 oz) of wine. Yet for that daily ration he drew from a decent variety of fare, such as mutton, veal, partridge, fish, broths, bread and *panado*, a sweet bread soup. The only foods that Cornaro did not allow himself to consume were tree fruits, because the classical physicians had warned they were difficult to digest.

The shed weight and restored vigour convinced Cornaro that, as he put it, 'healthy hunger was a constant and natural companion of a moderate lifestyle.'[38] He justified his conclusion in terms that any ancient Greek physician would have understood, writing that 'nature, desirous to preserve man in good health as long as possible, informs him, herself, how he is to act in time of illness.'[39] Nature communicates this by withdrawing the ill individual's hunger 'in order that he may eat but little'. The message served to remind Cornaro that 'nature . . . is satisfied with little', and he took the first step to recovery by acting with this in mind.[40] For Cornaro the body contained the wisdom for preserving itself in fine fettle through long years. If an individual might only learn to heed that wisdom, he might, Cornaro believed, 'become his own Physician'.[41]

Cornaro became his own physician and lived to the ripe old age of 82 years. He spent his extended second act travelling, visiting with his grandchildren and reading. He also stumped for a Hippocratic approach to health in which brief fasts played a central role. He wasn't troubled that any such return to pre-Christian medicine involved disentangling fasting from concerns about the hereafter, instead recalling to the popular consciousness fasting's benefits in the here and now. A strict Catholic, Cornaro took care to point out that, whatever the benefits in the material world, a temperate diet was also 'agreeable to the Deity'.[42]

The classical medical revival spearheaded by Cornaro did not endure much beyond his time, long though it was. The next two centuries would see fasting continue to be more of a religious practice than a health practice.

Cornaro's rescue from oblivion came courtesy of Christoph Wilhelm Hufeland (1762–1836), personal physician to that towering figure of German letters Johann Wolfgang von Goethe. So taken was Hufeland by Cornaro's idea of patient as physician that he penned and published *Macrobiotics: The Art of Prolonging Life* (1796). In this work, Hufeland innovated on the classical system of medicine by claiming that individuals are ill more or less all the time. In his view, only a wholesome environment, exercise and a temperate diet – Hufeland advocated a vegetarian one – kept people from becoming outright invalids. In fact, he went so far as to insist that 'light, heat, and oxygen are the real proper nourishment and sustenance of the vital power.'[43] He believed too that fasting could cure various ills, and cited as evidence a report of a military officer who was purported to have lost his sanity yet was restored to his wits by the practice.[44]

Hufeland took as his own Cornaro's conviction that sound health followed from allowing nature to run its course. As it turned out, Hufeland's writing, which revived classical medicine for the modern age, would contribute to a school of thought many would turn to for a rather interesting reason.

Relief from Doctors

That reason, in a nutshell, was relief from doctors. Not relief *from* doctors, mind you. Relief from *doctors*. Hufeland's *Macrobiotics* appeared in print amid a vogue for an aggressive approach to medicine. This approach had been born in seventeenth-century France. Its practitioners earned the epithet 'heroic' because they were said to show courage in administering their treatments, which were so extreme as to be nearly fatal. (Of the heroism of patients who underwent the treatments little is written.) Like their classical predecessors, these doctors agreed on the medical fundamentals of bodily humours and the imbalance thereof as the source of all illness and indisposition. Unlike their predecessors, however, they scorned dietetics and a holistic approach. Humoral balance could not be restored simply by allowing nature to do its work. Rather, they maintained that it came only in response to jolts and insults to the body. Heroic physicians thus plied their patients with violent purgatives and emetics, bled them and fed them mercury – all in a bid to draw out excess fluids and set the patient on the path to recovery. You could be sure that any fasts recommended by these doctors would carry you to the brink of death before you ever set foot on that path.

Heroic medicine touched individuals of every station, joining king and commoner in equal misery with its application. A single year saw France's Louis XIII (1601–1643) endure 212 enemas, 215 vomiting sessions and 47 bloodlettings. His successor, famed 'Sun King' Louis XIV (1638–1715), would receive over 2,000 enemas – sometimes four in a day – before night fell on his earthly reign. Ordinary French subjects had at their disposal *limonadiers du posterior* ('lemonade-makers of the ass'), their fond name for pharmacists who specialized in mixing and administering enemas.[45] Across the Atlantic, physicians attending George Washington (1732–1799) took an approach to treating their patient that was altogether in keeping with the times. The first u.s. president spent his final days being bled repeatedly, wrapped in plasters dosed with cantharidin (a poisonous secretion of the blister beetle) and given mercury chloride. The heroic treatments were to no avail, alas, and the Revolutionary War hero died on 14 December 1799.

Unsurprisingly, the public grew leery of such treatments and the 'heroic' physicians behind them. Distrust drove a search for alternatives, and there to serve as one was Hufeland's medical system. Its gentler therapies soon inspired others to develop alternatives of their own.

A therapy developed by Vincent Priessnitz (1799–1851), a semi-literate Austrian peasant, was based on water's healing powers. Priessnitz became convinced of these powers, having observed a roebuck heal a wounded leg by dipping it in a pond. When a baling accident injured Priessnitz's arm and broke two of his ribs, he attempted a version of the roebuck's cure. Unfazed by the fact that he had been told his case was hopeless, Priessnitz drank lots of water and bound wet bandages to his chest with dry ones. Before long he was as good as new. The routine became known as the Priessnitz Compress and from it he elaborated an entire system of natural healing that he called 'hydrotherapy'.[46]

Hydrotherapy became something of an industry, as folks from all over came to Priessnitz for bandaging, bathing and sweats. With its blend of Hippocratic and Galenic medicine, eighteenth-century French philosopher Jean-Jacques Rousseau's back-to-nature ethic, and mysticism, Priessnitz's system helped to foster a young but growing natural cure movement.

Natural Cure Practitioners

Fasting did not initially have a very significant role in the therapeutics of early natural cure practitioners. Hufeland advocated a moderate diet of light fare and Priessnitz fed his patients meat and dark bread. But as theories of natural healing evolved and more treatments arrived on the scene, fasting's role in the emerging practice grew greater.

The United States – which, along with Germany, was a seedbed for the movement – saw fasting grow in prominence as early as 1822. That year a Yale-educated physician named Isaac Jennings (1788–1874) reportedly took into his care a young woman suffering from typhoid fever. He became convinced that her case was hopeless, ended her treatment and left her to fast on spring water. Astonishingly, the young woman recovered. The reversal in prognosis upended Jennings's faith in heroic medical practices. From then on, in place of drugs he prescribed rest, exercise, exposure to sunlight, a vegetarian diet and occasional fasts. Though his approach later came under the names of 'orthopathy' and 'natural hygiene', Jennings, with fitting Yankee plainness, contented himself to call it his 'Let-alone Plan'.[47]

Jennings did not stand alone in his rejection of heroic medicine. His Let-alone Plan was inspired by the writings on health and hygiene by Sylvester Graham (1794–1851), the Presbyterian minister, diet reformer and inventor of the sweetish cracker that to this day bears his name. Graham frequently advocated fasts in his *Graham Journal of Health and Longevity*. When properly supervised and accompanied by bathing and the inevitable enemas, 'fasting removes those substances which are of the least use to the economy', Graham wrote, 'and hence all morbid accumulations, such as wens, tumors, abscesses and so on, are rapidly diminished and often wholly removed.'[48] The German hydrotherapist Benedict Lust (1872–1945) echoed Graham's belief, calling fasting a 'bloodless operation.'[49] (Lust also enjoys the distinction of having coined the term 'naturopath', a label which he attached to himself and practitioners like him and which is still in use today.)

Allopathic Medicine

By the middle of the nineteenth century the natural cure movement had gained purchase enough in the United States to pose a serious challenge to conventional medicine. The latter's practitioners feared that the growing popularity of alternative therapies would knock them from their dominant status, their approach relegated to simply one among many to choose from. This fear was not unfounded: the naturopaths had done much to promote such thinking in patients' minds by coining the label 'allopathic physicians', which served to highlight conventional medical practitioners' limited signature offerings of drugs and surgery.[50]

It became clear to these allopathic physicians, then, that they must seize the initiative while they could. Happily for them, they occupied a rather fortified position, thanks to the many schools, professional societies and publications they had founded. In 1842, they formed the American Medical Association, a professional body conjured into being, as its charter read, 'for the protection of their interests, for the maintenance of their honour and respectability, for the advancement of their knowledge, and the extension of their usefulness'.[51] They also created a code of medical ethics, standardized medical education and gave real teeth to state licensure requirements by filing charges against unlicensed healers of every stripe.

Through these assets, the practitioners of allopathic medicine exerted considerable influence – influence which they harnessed to foment public distrust of their naturopathic rivals. They mounted a propaganda campaign larded with both smear and fear tactics. They referred to natural healers as 'irregulars', a disparaging label meant to emphasize a lack of scientific rigour (whereas in truth early allopathic medicine could boast of no greater rigour); and they characterized fasting, which was by this time a familiar natural therapy, as dangerously unproven.

Natural healers and their allies pushed back against this propaganda assault, especially as it touched on fasting. One proponent lamented: 'The physiology of fasting in time of sickness is so entirely new to the medical world that every death that occurs with those who practice it is certain to be attributed to starving.'[52] Natural-healing true believers spilled much ink, in books and editorials, with the aim of debunking claims of the therapy's deadliness.

Henry Tanner

One man believed that words weren't enough. What was needed was an act, one to prove that an individual may not only survive a fast for far longer than ten days, but also benefit from it.

That man was the flamboyant Ohio physician Henry Tanner (1831–1918). Tanner had long held an interest in natural healing. In 1859 he received his degree from the Eclectic Medical Institute of Cincinnati. The institute taught a peculiarly North American form of naturopathy involving physical therapy and native botanicals; it deemed these cures preferable to synthetic drugs. As a practitioner Tanner came to regard fasting as a desirable therapy as well, believing that it could succeed where conventional medicine had failed.

Tanner occasionally carried his belief to extremes. He once forced his wife, who had fallen ill, to eat close to 1.5 kilograms (3 lb) of green beans a day. When the beans failed to alleviate her symptoms, he switched her to turnips. Shortly after this, she left him.[53]

Tanner's over-the-top approach to healing, though detrimental to his personal life, proved a boon to the natural cure movement. In 1877, he fell ill with what he described as 'low gastric fever'.[54] He resolved to forgo eating until his symptoms subsided. After ten days his symptoms had vanished, and he felt markedly better. Still, determined to prove the body could thrive without food, he continued to fast. His colleagues tried to turn him from what they thought was a suicidal course. 'The case continued without material change until the forty-first day,' wrote a colleague

whom Tanner tasked with supervising his fast. 'I became
alarmed at his condition, and strenuously urged him to
endeavor to allay the gastric irritation by taking considerable
quantities of milk.'[55] This Tanner did, and soon followed it
with a few crackers, breaking his fast. Despite having not
eaten for over a month, he was none the worse. Even more
impressively, he was cured of his ailment. Word soon spread,
and Tanner's fast was featured in newspapers throughout the
United States.

His allopathic colleagues, however, remained sceptical.
They wanted him to fast under more controlled and scientific
conditions. Neurologist William Hammond (1828–1900)
even promised to give him $1,000 if he succeeded – and
a decent burial if he didn't. Tanner was game. 'The task
before me', he said, 'is to negative (if possible) the hypothesis
laid down by my professional brethren and others that a
total abstinence from food for forty-two days, without a
suspension of the vital principle, is an impossibility.'[56]

It was with this goal in mind that, at the stroke of noon on
28 June 1880, Tanner began what he hoped would become a
month-long fast. He prepared simply by drinking a quart of
milk for breakfast and another at 11:45 a.m. Then he stripped
and permitted his person and clothing to be searched for
any hidden food. The same was done to the bed he was to
sleep in. He was weighed (71.4 kg/157½ lb) and measured
(101 cm/40 in. at the breast, 98.4 cm/38¾ in. at the abdomen,
55.9 cm/22 in. at the thigh and 29.2 cm/11½ in, at mid-arm).
His pulse, temperature and respiration were all normal.

Few besides a handful of the institute's faculty witnessed
Tanner's fast the first week, but word of it quickly spread,

drawing other curious physicians as well as the press. The *New York Herald* reporters staked out the institution lest they miss any detail of Tanner's progress. That progress was marked by highs and lows, even in the early going. Three days in he was asked if his appetite had acquired an edge. 'Oh! Yes; I feel a hunger, but I don't allow it to get the better of me,' came his reply. 'I keep it under the control of my will.'[57]

Yet his will could not master everything. On the fifth day he felt poorly. His pulse had dropped. Already he had shed 4.5 kilograms (10 lb). Despite this decline in well-being Tanner was suspected of somehow smuggling in food. One physician claimed to have seen him given something by a friend on the tenth day of his fast: a sponge possibly soaked in beef tea. It turned out that Tanner had in fact been slipped a sponge, but it was moistened only with water.

Tanner's fast was marked by highs and lows. One day might find him spirited; another, agitated or sulky. He kept up his strength with walks around the hall of his residence at the college or with drives through Central Park. Deep into his fast he would often vomit mucus and bile. He took this in stride, however, insisting that it was to be expected. It could be said of him that for the most part he bore his starvation without complaint.

Such remarkable stoicism electrified thousands, thanks to the extensive press coverage it received. Tanner was inundated with letters from people the world over. A group of students from Spain paid him a visit to serenade him. Sceptics came to poke and prod him. Men read books to him. A woman proposed.

After 42 days, Tanner ended his fast with much ceremony. A crowd had gathered to witness him do so. From it stepped forth a young child to present him with a peach. Tanner announced that he would eat the peach at the stroke of noon. A nearby factory whistle shrilled. Tanner bit into the fruit. The crowd cheered. One physician stepped to a piano and played a rousing air. Tanner finished his peach, waved a handkerchief and drank some soured milk. A second cheer erupted from the crowd. Never, he declared, had milk tasted so good. On seeing a large Georgia watermelon being trundled Tanner's way, a few onlooking physicians protested that it would prove too much. 'You let me alone,' Tanner rejoined. 'I have been through this before, and I know the condition of my stomach better than anyone else,' and adding for good measure, 'You are governed by theory, while I judge from experience.'[58] With these words he fell on the watermelon, devouring most of it.

Tanner ended his fast 16.3 kilograms (36 lb) lighter and quite a bit weaker than he began it. Otherwise, he was unharmed – though it was remarked that his 'blood corpuscles' had had a 'ragged appearance' on examination.[59] (The reason for this appearance is unknown, though red blood cells can take on a ragged appearance as they age.) Ample steak, apples, potatoes stewed in milk, beef tea, Hungarian wine and English ale soon restored him to full vigour. Three days after ending his fast, Tanner returned to his usual occupations.

New Varieties of Fasts

The hoopla surrounding Tanner's exploit brought fasting to public awareness as a viable alternative to conventional treatments, many of which were invasive, sickness-inducing in their own right or otherwise quite unpleasant. And so many followed his example. On the very same day that Tanner began his highly publicized fast, Agnes Dehart, a 21-year-old woman from Staten Island, New York, undertook her own in a bid to cure her stomach ulcers.[60] Various ills likewise prompted a band of fasters in Whanganui, New Zealand, to spend thirty days of the year 1907 living solely on orange juice.[61] And Horace Fletcher (1849–1919), originator of the thorough-chewing method known as 'Fletcherizing', claimed that a water fast of two or three weeks would cure rheumatism.[62]

As interest in fasting for health grew, so too did the varieties of fasts you could undertake. Some were clearly absurd and, worse, heedless of the age-old call to moderation. Others, however, in their restraint prefigured the fasts advocated by some medical practitioners today.

Arnold Ehret (1866–1922), a German émigré to the United States, developed one of the more offbeat approaches to fasting. His family had been plagued by illness (his father and brother had died of tuberculosis and his mother suffered from kidney disease), and Ehret decided that conventional cures were largely useless. He too suffered from kidney and heart disease and found little relief from various treatments and special diets. Finally, while on a trip to Algiers, he stopped eating altogether. He was surprised to find his health vastly improved, so much so that he followed his fast

with a 1,600-kilometre (1,000 mi.) bicycling trip. When
he returned, he devoted himself to studying the practice.

Ehret's erudition would culminate in his Mucusless Diet
Healing System, which he developed in the 1920s. The system
rested on his theory of pus- and mucus-forming foods as
the cause of various ills, constipation being the worst of
them. The Mucusless Diet Healing System forbade the consumption of meat, dairy, eggs and most grains and legumes,
because Ehret believed that they spurred the formation of
white blood cells, which in turn produced mucus and pus.[63]
Only foods that did not promote the formation of these
bodily fluids – fruits, nuts and leafy greens, to name a few –
would restore a sufferer to health.

Ehret would also recommend regular fasts. In fact, he
believed the body did not require food at all: it was akin to an
air-gas engine, and food served only to jam its workings. (We
hear in this echoes of Hufeland's own notion that light, heat
and air were a body's ideal sustenance.) Ehret's entire system
merely elaborated a simple equation, 'Vitality = Power –
Obstruction', which is perhaps why it later captivated a
teenaged Steve Jobs. The Apple founder and CEO followed
the system until his death, in 2011.

Those unconvinced of mucus and pus's uniformly evil
roles in poor health could seek other inventive fasts, such
as the one devised by an American abroad, Norman Walker
(1886–1985). The sight of a French peasant peeling carrots
inspired him to begin a carrot juice delivery service in
California. Subsisting on fresh juices, nuts and seeds would
prevent constipation, 'the primary cause of nearly every
disturbance of the human system,' he claimed.[64]

John Henry Tilden (1851–1940) would place blame on supposedly toxic metabolic waste, the accumulation of which he thought caused illness. In 1914 he established a sanitarium where patients could rid themselves of toxic waste through fasting and other therapies. And corpulent business tycoon turned health food advocate Henry Lindlahr (1862–1924) would preach a gospel of health inspired by the Priessnitzian water cures. In 1914 he established his own institute devoted to natural therapies.

As the nineteenth century drew to a close, interest in therapeutic fasts began to extend beyond the naturopathic strongholds of Germany and the United States. Thanks to influence from American practitioners, in the United Kingdom a 'natural cure' movement took hold – one that exalted exercise, a diet of whole foods, fresh air and positive thinking as the keys to health and well-being. The first natural cure clinic opened in Edinburgh, Scotland, in 1938. It was followed by clinics in Buckinghamshire and Hertfordshire in England. Among other treatments, these clinics offered therapeutic fasting of a few days to three months.

Meanwhile in Germany, great strides were made in scientific validation of fasting's virtues, which had been a goal since Tanner's time. This progress came by way of the physician Otto Buchinger (1878–1966), who was the first to document convincingly fasting's remedial effects on disease. His findings were such that they led him to declare fasting 'the most effective biological treatment'.[65] In words reminiscent of his earlier countryman Benedict Lust, Buchinger added: 'It is the operation without surgery.'[66] Buchinger would go on to open several clinics where patients fasted on juices for weeks at a time.

Buchinger's endorsement of fasting as a cure-all did not, however, make much of an impact outside Germany. The allopathic camp was making strides of its own – strides that would leave natural cures in the dust for some time. Such drug breakthroughs as sulfa, penicillin and Jonas Salk's polio vaccine captured the public's imagination, which, as it turned out, was key to winning its loyalty. People once again began to look to pharmaceuticals for cures. The zeitgeist of the twentieth-century post-war period clearly favoured allopathy, and its practitioners lost no time in once again levelling charges of scientific indiscipline at their naturopathic rivals.

The latter contingent, meanwhile, had done itself no favours. Quacks began to outnumber and overshadow their more grounded peers, an unfortunate development that only added weight and substance to accusations cast at the whole of the profession. Naturopathy did not die, exactly, nor did the practice of fasting. Their appeal, however, did become largely limited to various bohemian and countercultural circles at the fringes of society. At any rate, it no longer posed the threat to allopathy that it had in decades past. Conventional medicine reigned supreme.

This was certainly a bitter pill for natural healers to swallow.

Re-emergence of Fasting

This reign would not continue unchallenged. In the closing decades of the twentieth century, conventional medicine came to confront the fact that certain health problems defied pharmaceutical solutions. No pill, for instance, could cure obesity or its associated metabolic disorders. Interest in possible treatments thus began to range beyond what could be gleaned from the *Physician's Desk Reference*. And there all along had been fasting.

Fast-forward to 2017 and Jeanette Winterson's stay at the Buchinger Wilhelmi Clinic. Today there are hundreds of such clinics the world over offering fasts for a range of illnesses. Some of those fasts are dedicated entirely to slimming, as we'll see in the next chapter.

4

SEEING LESS OF YOU: THE PROMISE OF FASTING FOR WEIGHT LOSS

'Men and women of the first social importance have fasted and rolled on the floor in calisthenic contortions. Perhaps they have triumphed in a measure; perhaps they have gone forth to table with a more awful and more formidable appetite. The tragedy of fat!'
– Vance Thompson[1]

Twenty-seven-year-old Angus Barbieri (1939–1990) just wanted a woman to share his life. 'I never had a steady girl,' he said. 'Being so fat, I was far too shy to ask for a date.'[2] In 1965 the Scotsman, who had spent most of his adulthood working in his family's fish and chip shop, checked himself into Dundee's Maryfield Hospital. The condition that brought him there was his weight, which had reached 207 kilograms (456 lb).

The hospital stay proved sobering and transformative. From that day on Barbieri observed a radically overhauled diet, living on nothing but coffee, soda water and vitamins. He felt no worse for the change, and often did chores around the hospital. 'I got up each morning and then helped with the work in the ward,' he said of his stay. 'I even did some cooking. I had a reputation as a good cook, working in my father's family fish and chips shop, and I wanted to show my will power against eating.'[3] In this he succeeded admirably. His fast lasted 382 days. He broke it with a breakfast of one boiled egg and some bread with butter. 'It went down OK,' he said of this first meal in over year. 'I feel a bit full, but I thoroughly enjoyed it.'[4]

During his stay at Maryfield Hospital Angus managed to lose 133 kilograms (294 lb). In time, he also found love, got married and had two sons. With greater personal fulfilment came recognition. He was awarded a Guinness World Record for longest fast and became something of a media sensation. Such notoriety was all well and good, but his most important and lasting contribution was to the science of nutrition. He showed that fasting could effectively combat obesity.

Angus Barbieri exemplified how, under the right conditions and for the right reasons, human beings can bear up under fasting conditions for extended periods of time. We know also from the Minnesota Starvation Experiment and other investigations that fasting diets can often yield unexpected benefits. Perhaps the most dismaying takeaway of all, however – that a semi-starvation diet is a difficult undertaking – bred in even determined dieters a fatalistic attitude. This attitude extended to the physicians caring for these dieters. 'Many obese persons today might well be better off if they learned to live with their condition, and stopped subjecting themselves over and over to painful and frustrating attempts to lose weight,' psychiatrist and eating disorder treatment pioneer Albert Stunkard (1922–2014) told attendees of Richard Nixon's White House Conference on Food, Nutrition and Health in 1969.[5]

The feat pulled off by Barbieri thus seemed all more astonishing. The stalwart Scot went without eating for a solid year, and whatever pangs of hunger he experienced in that time failed to deter him. It turned out that he had a little help in staving off those pangs.

Ketosis

That help came from within. In the late 1950s, a few years before Barbieri checked into Maryfield Hospital, Walter Lyon Bloom, physician and director of medical education and research at Piedmont Hospital in Atlanta, Georgia, undertook a series of extensive studies of fasting's effect on obesity. In one of the most fruitful of those studies, he recruited nine subjects with obesity. The subjects were both male and female, and each had experienced trouble in past dieting attempts. Bloom nonetheless trusted that the appetite-quashing power of ketosis, a unique state in which the body sought fuel in its own fat and protein, might aid them in losing weight. To this end, he tasked them with fasting for four to nine days. It turned out that each of his study's participants experienced enough of a reduction in appetite that they were able to prevail in their fasts. (Bloom encouraged his subjects to quit should they experience discomfort.)

One male subject found fasting so easy and efficacious that he extended his fast to eighteen days. Yet even those of Bloom's subjects who ended their fasts after a week saw lasting effects. They were satisfied by portions that were smaller than they were used to, and they felt no envy when eating with people who were given larger portions.[6] Best of all, they lost about 1.2 kilograms (2.7 lb) a day. Even after the study ended, they either continued to lose weight by following a reducing diet or they maintained their weight.[7]

Both fasting and carbohydrate restriction made hunger all but disappear. Faced with limited resources under such conditions, the body entered ketosis, and the resulting satiety helped the subjects achieve their weight loss goals, Bloom concluded.[8] Ketosis turned out to be a highly effective diet aid.

The metabolic phenomenon of ketosis gained added validity when studies after Bloom's own were carried out a few years later at the University of California, Los Angeles, and yielded many of the same results. Patients with obesity, eleven in all, spent anywhere from twelve to 117 days starving. Through this period of starvation, to researchers' surprise, the participants felt little hunger. Their experience stood in stark contrast to earlier reports of 'hunger and suffering' from 'individuals who, over a prolonged period, consume a calorically inadequate diet'.[9] Outright fasting, rather than dieting, revealed itself to be the easiest treatment for obesity. What's more, as the editors of the *Journal of the American Medical Association* noted, 'gratifying weight loss without hunger may bring about the desired immediate results and help establish a normal eating pattern where other dietary restrictions fail'.[10] Fasting bolstered dieters' confidence in their ability to control their eating.

Ketosis seemed to physicians a potentially foolproof way to treat obesity. In 1887 German researcher Eduard Külz first noted the byproducts of ketosis in the urine of a psychotic patient who went without food for three days.

Another physician noted them in the urine of a woman who had refused all food. He found that when he gave her even a small amount of sugar, the ketones – acids that result when the body breaks down fat for energy – disappeared. Soon physicians all over were noting the presence of ketone bodies in fasting patients. One physician noted the presence of ketones in Giovanni Succi's urine, having succeeded where Francis Gano Benedict failed by managing to study the famous hunger artist. The concentration increased each passing day until it eventually levelled out after 28 days.[11] Benedict himself took part in the trend, detecting ketone bodies in the urine of his subject, the inimitable Agostino Levanzin whom we met in Chapter Two.

The ketone bodies observed in the urine of these fasting men were of three kinds: ss-Hydroxybutyric acid, acetoacetate and acetone. (This last ketone body is the same chemical found in nail polish remover.) All are produced in the liver from fatty acids.[12] These ketone bodies are water soluble and therefore able to cross the blood–brain barrier, which allows them to serve as fuel for the brain in the absence of glucose.[13] When this crossing happens, the body is in a state of ketosis.

Ketosis, a biochemical adaptation that enables a person to fast for months, allowed Angus Barbieri to go a long time without food and suffer no fatal effect. His body never needed to resort to consuming the heart for his brain's nourishment. (Go without water, however, the element that is necessary for biochemical reactions to happen, and you'll live a mere three to four days.)

When you fast, you know you've entered ketosis when you notice certain telltale signs. You'll notice subtle changes in your body's sensations and odour, including breath that smells of nail polish remover, an odour brought on by ketones leaving your body through your respiration. You'll notice rapid weight loss, though, at first, most of it water weight. And you'll experience a dulled or reduced appetite.

'I hadn't eaten for the past 18 hours and I didn't even realize it,' reported one person on Reddit, a popular social media platform, regarding this last effect.[14] 'I have been on keto for almost two years and I feel free from food dominating my plans,' declared another user on the same thread: 'I can easily go for hours without eating.'[15] The effect of a dulled or reduced appetite explains the appeal of ketogenic diets. It makes them easier to follow than other diet methods.

Later research confirmed findings of earlier studies, as well as individual experience: ketogenic diets prevent an increase in ghrelin, the hormone that creates a sense of hunger and increases food intake.[16] Even more promising, it was found that ketosis can also mitigate the cognitive impairment caused by weight gain and have an overall beneficial effect on mood.[17] And when people in ketosis exercise, they oxidize – or burn – more fat.[18]

Although outright fasting is a sure way of achieving ketosis, a low-carbohydrate, semi-starvation diet also delivers results. In 1931, researchers placed 187 obese patients on a diet of 400 to 600 calories for almost nine weeks. They found the subjects lost an average of 1.6 kilograms (3½ lb) a week. Even more important, they felt great while doing so, reporting an increased sense of well-being, a decrease in fatigue and the disappearance of such minor ailments as headache and skin disorders.[19] A similar report of feeling great came from one 32-year-old Russian housewife after being placed on a semi-starvation diet of 600 calories and 35 grams (1.23 oz) of carbohydrate a day, which she followed for nine months.[20] To her delight, she stripped 108 kilograms (239 lb) from her 179 kilogram (395 lb) frame. Through the whole of her diet, the Russian woman claimed to have felt neither hunger nor weakness.[21]

Dangers and Side Effects of Ketogenic Diets

Such success stories made ketosis-inducing fasts the medical establishment's favoured treatment for obesity. Not all patients, however, experienced desirable effects. Indeed, some of them experienced the worst effect of all. In 1969, researchers reported the death of a twenty-year-old British woman.[22] Overweight since childhood, she weighed 118 kilograms (260 lb) when she came to a hospital in Southampton for treatment. Weight concerns aside, the young woman was otherwise healthy. The thirty-week fast that her doctors prescribed for her, which consisted of nothing except water and supplements, caused her to lose around 227 grams (0.5 lb) every day. Once she reached her ideal weight of 60 kg (132 lb), her doctors placed her on a low-carbohydrate, low-calorie refeeding diet. It seemed to agree with her; she felt and looked well, her blood pressure and other vitals were normal. She did suffer mild edema in her legs, but her physicians assumed it was benign and continued the refeeding. For the first two days, she was given 200 calories of protein and fat; the subsequent two days saw that allotment increased by another 200 calories, and so on.

On the seventh day of refeeding the newly slimmed patient said she felt faint. She went to bed, and shortly thereafter became unconscious and pale. Still, her blood pressure and pulse remained normal. The next morning she felt well again. Shortly after a breakfast of one egg, however, she suffered a heart attack, lost consciousness, stopped breathing and grew pale. With a closed-chest cardiac massage she came around again, only to suffer a second arrest seven hours later. Cardiac massage was applied once more, with success. But the next morning she had her final – and fatal – heart attack.

Her autopsy report showed 'gross destruction of cardiac myofibrils', long, fine fibres found in striated muscle cells.[23] Her physicians were flummoxed. They compared her damaged heart to a heart taken from a recently deceased woman with anorexia. Though the latter woman had starved herself for ten years, her heart showed no damage like that sustained by the heart of the newly dead fasting patient. To the question of what could account for the damage that occurred during a thirty-week fast in an otherwise healthy young woman physicians had no answer. They suggested only 'that this regimen should no longer be recommended as a safe means of weight reduction'.[24]

Though ketogenic dieters rarely died, they could experience other side effects, the severity of which ranged from merely unpleasant to quite serious. In the early 1960s physician Ernst J. Drenick (1916–1993) fasted ten men and one woman. The eleven patients ranged in age from 32 to 71 and in weight from 109 kilograms (240 lb) to 204 kilograms (450 lb). He found that their response to fasting varied significantly. All of them reported little to no hunger pangs, thanks to having entered a state of ketosis. Most remained energetic, and all lost significant amounts of weight. Some, however, developed orthostatic hypotension, or a pronounced decrease in blood pressure. They felt faint upon rising from bed and sometimes extremely weak as well. The sole woman in the study suffered acute arthritis (gout) in her left ankle.[25] Four patients became anaemic.

In his write-up of the study, which was printed in the *Journal of the American Medical Association*, Drenick was quick to acknowledge the benefits of the fast. He was astonished at how 'prolonged starvation was tolerated' (one of his patients happily fasted 117 days), which he attributed to ketosis. He also noted that, after the fast, many of the patients' eating habits and appetite 'seemed to have undergone a decisive change'.[26] Follow-up visits revealed his patients as having little difficulty maintaining their weight.

It was fast becoming clear that fasting diets did work. 'Complete abstinence from caloric consumption would appear to be the best approach,' Drenick concluded, his reason being that 'most seriously overweight patients are no longer capable of performing the physical exercises which would result in a significant expenditure of calories.'[27] Side effects did occur, not a few of which were concerning. Nonetheless, research sped apace on how to avoid the worst of them.

Supplemental Protein

Many physicians determined that the solution to these side effects was supplemental protein. Just what kind of supplemental protein suited best came under debate. The participants in this debate fell into two camps. Members of the first camp favoured protein from natural sources, such as poultry, fish and beef. Members of the second camp, meanwhile, favoured chemically defined protein, such as powders and shakes.

Dr George Blackburn (1936–2017) of the Center for Nutritional Research at New England Deaconess Hospital belonged to the first camp. He placed obese patients on fasts lasting anywhere from four to eleven months. Blackburn's prescribed fasts didn't demand full abstinence from his patients; they were granted each day about 227 grams (8 oz) of protein in the form of broiled fish, lean beef and poultry. The calories delivered by the supplemental protein did not, however, prevent Blackburn's patients from entering ketosis. They experienced few hunger pangs and lost impressive amounts of weight, often in excess of 45 kilograms (100 lb). Most importantly, they suffered no adverse effects.[28]

Physicians who championed chemically defined protein, meanwhile, thought the prospect of broiling fish and chicken too daunting for patients. Shakes were easier – if not tastier – and would prove more popular. They were right. In 1971, Mt Sinai Hospital in New York City saw four hundred patients actively enrolled in a protein-sparing liquid fast. Five times a day the participants treated themselves to a mixture of glucose, amino acids and minerals.[29]

Another member of the chemically defined-protein camp was American osteopath Robert Linn (1934–1998). Like the allopathic physicians at Mt Sinai Hospital, Linn thought chemical slurries the way to a dieter's heart. His 'Last Chance

Diet', created in the mid-1970s, had patients gulping Prolinn, a syrup of hydrolyzed collagen for mixing in water or diet soda. The concoction, which had a dreadful taste, delivered a mere 400 calories a day. Linn acknowledged that his diet seemed 'extreme', as he put it, but was quick to add that it responded to an extreme 'need of losing weight' felt by the individuals who adopted it.[30] Reportedly, the diet bred results that were just as extreme in terms of success. One satisfied customer marvelled at his own reduction, claiming that he shed '42 pounds [19 kg] in nine weeks', a rate that, as he described it, 'blows your mind'.[31]

Such enthusiasm belied some serious demerits. Linn's foul-tasting drink lacked essential vitamins, minerals and electrolytes. And, in a stroke of terrible luck, publication of the book on the diet, *The Last Chance Diet* (1977), happened to coincide with a warning, issued by the u.s. Food and Drug Administration, of the dangers of liquid diets. Sixteen women died of heart attacks and strokes, fatalities that the warning attributed to the fact that they had been following liquid diets at the time of their demise.[32] One physician speculated that the cardiac irregularities owed to potassium depletion, which can interfere with the normal electrical impulses in the heart.[33] In the report, Prolinn was named as one of the culprits. And the hits just kept on coming: a few years later, Linn found himself a defendant in a $4 million malpractice suit prompted by a patient's death fourteen days into the diet.[34]

Despite the dangers, not to mention the negative publicity, many felt that chemically defined protein was too lucrative a product to abandon. Physicians went back to the drawing board, and a decade later two of them, again in the employ of Mt Sinai Hospital, emerged with a new product. Like Prolinn, the Optifast Supplemental Fasting Program developed by Victor Vertes (1927–2014) and Saul Genuth (1931–2020) offered patients an unpleasant-tasting shake to drink five times a day. Yet it delivered results that were anything but unpleasant. Eighty per cent of Vertes and Genuth's Optifast patients lost at least 18 kilograms (40 lb) a month, with an average weight loss of about 38.5 kilograms (85 lb) by the diet's completion.[35] Even better, Optifast provided essential nutrients that had been missing in earlier protein drinks; as such, patients did not experience dangerous side effects.

But that didn't mean liquid protein diets were a silver bullet. As media mogul Oprah Winfrey discovered when she lost 30 kilograms (67 lb) on Optifast, weight began piling on again shortly after dieters drank the final shake of their diet. 'Two weeks after I returned to real food, I was up 10 pounds,' she said. 'Since I wasn't exercising, there was nothing my body could do but regain the weight.'[36] Regain the weight she did – and then some. And Winfrey wasn't alone: some dieters saw up to 70 per cent of their pre-reduction weight return after they completed their protein-shake fast.

Such setbacks likely owed to dieters' lack of understanding of fasting's proper use. Fasting should, when used properly, be considered an occasion for a change in eating habits rather than a quick weight-loss solution. By quelling hunger pangs, a ketosis-inducing fast can help us recognize – and thereby resist – the siren song of our obesogenic environment. There's nothing like fasting to train our attention on how often and how much we are manipulated to eat.

Of course, standing in the way is the fact that steering clear of food for days requires steadfast dedication; rare are individuals who relish counting the ketone bodies in their urine. It comes as no surprise, then, that modern diets succeeded most when dieters found some support, be it medical supervision or, indeed, even confinement to a hospital. Although this is as it ought to have been, the fact remains that people have fasted for millennia to lose weight without the care of physicians and medical institutions. The fasts undertaken before the advent of modern medicine may have lacked scientific guidance, but they made up for this in the guidance of innate wisdom. Their results often proved quite effective.

Moderate Attitudes to Fasting

Fasting diets undertaken by our classical forebears were not nearly as punishing as the diets followed today – no dreary spooning-up of cabbage soup, no counting of calories. (Indeed, the latter activity was impossible, because humankind would not reach an understanding of calories for around another two thousand years.) Their diets were rather milder, consisting of moderate fasts and some form of exercise. Yet they weren't so mild as to lack occasional quirks. Hippocrates counselled patients to 'take no baths . . . sleep on a hard bed', and 'only eat once per day'.[37] He went on to say that the sole daily meal is best taken immediately after vigorous exercise. Dieters ought to still be panting from their exertions when they sit down to eat, though it's best that they take a moment to vomit first.

Writing a few centuries later, Galen dispensed with the retching, but he similarly insisted that moderate exercise was beneficial, especially when accompanied by massage and a diet of barley, game and vegetables.[38] The regimen 'reduced a huge fat fellow to a moderate size in a short time', Galen claimed in his treatise *On the Power of Foods* (*De alimentorum facultatibus, c.* 165–75 CE). The good doctor made his patient 'run every morning until he fell into a profuse sweat'.[39] Then, 'some hours after', Galen 'permitted him to eat freely', yet only of food 'which afforded but little nourishment'.[40]

Indeed, prescriptions for undue self-starvation or other masochistic exercises in self-denial were unheard of in classical antiquity. This is because the ancients saw obesity in a different light. Though Hippocrates and Galen both agreed that morbid obesity was harmful, neither saw the presence of fat itself as promoting disease. The overweight patient simply suffered from a phlegmatic constitution: that is, a constitution marked by an abundance of the bodily humour phlegm. His girth was not the cause of disease; rather, his propensity for gluttony was the root of the problem. Overeating produced a surfeit of humours and dampened the fires of life.[41] Proper diet and exercise would set the unbalanced body once again to rights.

Changing Attitudes to Excess Weight

Such a moderate attitude to obesity persisted throughout the Middle Ages. By the seventeenth century, however, excess weight began to be looked upon with suspicion by European and British scholars. The change in perception perhaps owed to greater numbers of heavier individuals, thanks to agricultural innovations that served to increase the food supply; or, what's likelier, it may have owed to the spread of new theories of nutrition and metabolism that we considered in the previous chapter. The humoral theory of medicine was on the wane, which meant that the presence of fat was no longer taken as signalling a preponderance of phlegm. The perceptual shift proved so much the worse for heavier individuals, as fat itself thenceforth came to be looked on as repulsive, if not malignant.

Through several decades of the seventeenth century, earnest scholars penned dissertations and disputations on fat – no fewer than 34, to be exact – and they concurred that there was nothing good to say about it.[42] Scholar Karl Christian Leisner deplored the Rubenesque figure idealized by the German peasantry, who associated it with health and abundance. In his 1683 dissertation on the topic, he wrote that these 'simple' folk failed to understand that fat was not beautiful. It betrayed, he argued, a gross morbidity, one in which veins were clogged with the stuff, causing asthma, sterility and stupidity.[43]

Chiming with Leisner's notions were those held by the English physician Thomas Short (1690–1772). He deemed fat to be 'an undesirable Load of useless and pernicious Matter'.[44] This last quality made itself evident in causing a body to putrefy, a process that subjected the burdened individual to swooning, palpitations and fainting.[45] His horror at the effects of corpulence disposed Short to cast a jaundiced eye on the obese people whom he encountered. A 'Monster in nature for bulk' was how he described one woman who weighed 227 kilograms (500 lb).[46] Nothing, in his estimation, could be worse than being fat.

The negative characterizations elaborated by Leisner, Short and others took hold. By the end of the eighteenth century, fatness had become inextricably associated with disease. Perhaps not at all coincidentally, around this time greater numbers of people began to experiment with dieting as a means of losing weight. And fasting promised to be the most effective diet of all. No longer solely the practice of would-be saints, writes scholar Sander Gilman, fasting transformed into 'dieting as a means of affecting the material body rather than providing some metaphysical relationship between the godhead and human beings'.[47]

From this point on, the historical record becomes peopled with men and women filled with a loathing for, and an obsession with starving down, their all-too-fleshy material bodies. 'Whatever be the quantity that a man eats,' the English writer Samuel Johnson (1709–1784) said, 'it is plain that if he is too fat, he has eaten more than he should have done.'[48] This was a sin of which he was often guilty, and he atoned by fasting 'from the Sunday's dinner to the Tuesday's dinner without any inconvenience'.[49] In this he was joined by the gourmand Jean Anthelme Brillat-Savarin (1755–1826), who knew that excess must be tempered by abstinence. He warned that if you ignored his advice to cut down on your portions, you would 'become ugly, and thick, and asthmatic, and finally die in your own melted grease'.[50]

George Cheyne (1671–1743) perhaps best exemplified the new concern with slimming. He struggled with his weight from infancy. His 'glands were lax, his solid parts feeble', writes historian Hillel Schwartz of Cheyne's childhood physique. Adulthood saw him no more robust. He was, as he confessed, 'excessively fat, short-breath'd, lethargick, and listless'.[51]

Happily, Cheyne was himself a physician, and so was familiar with the array of treatments available. He tried a vegetarian diet to little avail. He followed this with about a dozen other cures: vomiting, volatile salts, draughts of opium, calomel, nips of bitters, iron water – there seemed no end to the caustic liquids that Cheyne would swallow in the name of slimness. He succeeded only in irritating his liver and gallbladder.

Out of desperation, Cheyne fasted for six months, milk his only sustenance. The fast worked. He lost weight and felt better. But Cheyne was not one to resist temptation for long. No sooner did he end his fast than he began gorging on animal flesh, and 'thereby suddenly grew *plump, fat,* and *hale* to a Wonder; but indeed too fast'.[52] He grew to 204 kilograms (450 lb). And with the pounds came a whole host of afflictions: asthma, scorbutic ulcers and erysipelas (a bacterial infection of the skin).[53] Chastened, he once again began to observe an austere diet, this time of milk and vegetables. 'The thinner my diet is,' he wrote in 1733, 'the easier, more cheerful and lightsome I find myself.'[54]

Cheyne had made an important observation. Slimming need not involve starvation or caustic purgatives. A moderate fast could yield satisfactory results. As the eighteenth century ceded to the nineteenth, fasting diets abounded, at the same time lessening in severity to appeal to working men and women.

Alfred William Moore's Diet

One such gentler diet was that which British physician Alfred William Moore urged on his patients. It involved eating no food between 9:00 a.m. and 5:00 p.m., a practice that, as he wrote in 1857, must be 'scrupulously observed and adhered to' if it were to work.[55] Scrupulously observed as well should be the light, nourishing nature of the meals that bookended the fast. For breakfast Moore prescribed a serving of biscuit, not to exceed 57 grams (2 oz), one egg and two cups of coffee. Dinner should consist of more biscuit and a medley of vegetables – sea kale, spinach, carrots, turnips and other produce low in starch – along with 198 grams (7 oz) of meat. Hunger pangs late in the day could be driven away with gruel, a dish whose 'highly phosphoric principles' offset its starchiness, in a portion no greater than 227 grams (8 oz).[56] Other starchy foods, including bread, were forbidden, as was liquor; Moore thought them especially fattening.

Easy to follow and not terribly restrictive, Moore's diet became quite popular. And it produced some impressive successes, freeing a magistrate from his pot belly, slimming a young lady of short stature and so 'exceedingly fat that her head appeared buried in her shoulders' and reducing a clergyman of the Church of England whose post-marriage *embonpoint* caused him 'great annoyance', among others.[57]

Edward Hooker Dewey's No-Breakfast Plan

Across the Atlantic, Americans had grown keen on fasting cures. In 1900 the physician Edward Hooker Dewey

(1837–1904) introduced his No-Breakfast Plan, and it entailed exactly that. Dewey had observed that those patients of his who forewent meals regained their health more quickly than patients who did not. Eating when under the weather, it seemed, made an illness worse. Starve a patient, however, and he would soon be on the mend. 'In every case of recovery,' Dewey observed, 'there was a history of increasing general strength as the disease declined, of an actual increase of vital power without the support of food.'[58]

If fasting could cure the seriously ill, why not the mildly infirm? As he was mulling this question over, Dewey encountered a friend recently returned from Europe. 'At once he began to talk . . . about the exceedingly light breakfasts customary in all the great centres where he had been,' he wrote. 'They consisted only of a roll and a cup of coffee.'[59] This made sense to Dewey, for he noted that there was 'no natural hunger in the morning'.[60] Following the European example, he too swore off breakfast – which for him usually featured ham, sausage, eggs, steak and chops – in a bid to relieve his dyspepsia. His colleagues thought he had gone crazy. But Dewey felt quite the opposite. He grew thin, yes, but he also felt himself suffused with vigour and a sense of well-being. When he 'gave up all eating in the morning', Dewey claimed, it produced 'such reviving effects upon [his] powers that the results began to be noticed by all friends'.[61]

So energizing did Dewey find his no-breakfast regimen that he was moved to tell the world of its virtues. In 1900 he published *The No-Breakfast Plan and the Fasting-Cure*, which recommends to its readers regular fasts of eighteen hours in length.

Dewey's prescription drew both sceptics and adherents. Many still thought breakfast essential to good health. Yet others could not deny that skipping it rid them of indigestion and other ills. It was estimated that, in a single New England town, one hundred people followed Dewey's plan. A banker was said to have placed his family, servants and dog on two meals a day. A publisher claimed Dewey's system cured him of lung disease.[62]

Sceptics deemed Dewey crazy and, as he himself recounts, 'watched [his practice] with hostile interest, as if homicide from starvation were the inevitable result in all cases'.[63] It seemed he was watched – and criticized – wherever he went. In 1902 during a visit to England, Dewey held a lecture in Manchester, where *The Guardian* greeted him with a spate of sarcastic articles about Mancunians 'addicted to fads'.[64] A few years later, the *British Medical Journal* described Dewey as 'not an accurate or careful writer', and pointed out errors in his *No-Breakfast Plan*.[65]

Firm in his conviction that the true enemy of health was overindulgence, Dewey and his work weathered their scepticism with aplomb. *The No-Breakfast Plan* sold well and, by 1921, had seen four reprints and translations into German and French. And for good reason: Dewey's moderate regimen swiftly produced admirable results. Many quailed at the prospect of undertaking a prolonged fast or semi-starvation diet, yet skipping breakfast seemed eminently doable. The No-Breakfast Plan thus was a nice compromise, one that could whittle the waistline of even the most reluctant dieter.

Intermittent Fasting

Though few remember Dewey's name today, the spirit of his No-Breakfast Plan lives on in its present guise of intermittent fasting. Indeed, intermittent fasting is but one of a variety of brief fasts. You can, like Dewey, still skip breakfast and reap benefits. But you can also fast on alternate days (skipping eating every other day), periodically (forgoing food every few days) or during certain windows of time (skipping breakfast, lunch or dinner). Alternatively, you might fast in less clearly defined ways, subsisting on juice or, like Cheyne, milk.

All these variations yield benefits. One study showed that time-restricted feeding resulted in an average weight loss of 7 kilograms (15½ lb), most likely because participants were eating fewer calories.[66] Another study showed that time-restricted eating can cause one to lose weight even if dieters eat as many calories as they did before they embarked on their fasts. Researchers attributed this unexpected weight reduction to fasting's seeming ability to transform white fat into the more metabolically active brown fat.[67]

This ability to boost the metabolism means fasting can bestow benefits on the woefully unfit. In laboratory experiments fasting yielded more benefits for low-aerobic-capacity animals – that is, out-of-shape rats. Low-aerobic capacity is an undesirable state to be in, linked as it is to higher risk for metabolic-related diseases (type 2 diabetes, heart disease, stroke) and decreased longevity. And although traditional calorie-cutting does not have a marked effect on such individuals, the experiments found that intermittent fasting caused them to lose more weight than their leaner, fitter counterparts. Even more impressive was that the low-aerobic-capacity rats lost weight despite their low level of daily physical activity. The upshot? The same likely holds for humans as well, meaning intermittent fasting may be especially helpful for obesity-prone, unfit individuals.[68]

Studies on humans have been just as promising. Trials ranging from two to twelve weeks showed that intermittent fasting resulted in weight loss, regardless of changes in overall caloric intake. And there's plenty of anecdotal evidence that support these findings: in 2014, journalist Peter Bowes reported to the BBC on his experience with intermittent fasting. He lost weight and 'felt more alert a lot of the time'.[69] He also showed a drop in insulin-like growth factor, a hormone that has been linked to colorectal, breast and prostate cancer.[70] And The Guardian has changed its opinion of fasting since the days of Edward Hooker Dewey's No-Breakfast Plan. 'Fasting intermittently is incredibly effective when it comes to losing weight,' journalist Zoe Williams writes in the publication. 'On the days when I was fasting, I often had more energy and slept better.'[71] Such additional benefits likely do much to encourage people to follow the diet until they reach their goal weight.

Most of the benefits of intermittent fasting appear after you've fasted longer than twelve hours. Which twelve hours should you fast? Some scientists claim it is dinner rather than breakfast that we should be skipping. (But most agree that skipping any meal can provide great benefits.) Dinner, as a meal taken late in the day, disrupts the body's circadian rhythms, the 24-hour cycle of physiological processes to which all living creatures are subject.[72] These rhythms affect the functions of every aspect of our biology, including our gastrointestinal tract. As day turns to night, the gastrointestinal tract slows down (as we too slow down). There is a decrease in blood flow and gastric emptying (a process by which food moves from the stomach to the upper intestine), as well as in the body's response to glucose. Yet this relaxation does not mean the body isn't busy elsewhere: the select repose of certain organs and processes means the body can devote energy to general repair and rejuvenation.[73]

Eating at night disrupts this general slowdown. Evening fasts therefore return us to the body's natural rhythms. Dr Deborah Wexler, director of the Massachusetts General Hospital Diabetes Center, has noted that 'evidence [suggests] that the circadian rhythm fasting approach, where meals are restricted to an eight to 10-hour [sic] period of the daytime, is effective.' And its effectiveness rests on the idea that it is beneficial to your health to put food in your system when its mechanisms for dealing with it are their most active.[74]

A spate of recent studies supports the idea that intermittent fasting is a good way to try out fasting for those who wish to shed a few kilograms. Still, it bears mentioning that other studies have found intermittent fasting to bring about no more weight loss than a reduced-calorie diet.[75] Researchers randomized one hundred overweight and obese people in one of three groups – the first alternate-day fasting, the second a diet restricted to 75 per cent of regular daily caloric intake and the third a control group following a regular eating plan. They found that both the fasting and the calorie-restricted group had lost 6.8 per cent of their weight. After one year, the fasting group was down 6 per cent, and the calorie-restricted group 5.3 per cent. In other words, there was no statistical difference.[76] Even worse, the alternate-day fasting group had a higher dropout rate.

Still, for those who dislike traditional diets, fasting is worth trying. From extreme ketogenic fasts – which should only be done under a physician's guidance – to more moderate intermittent fasts, there is ample evidence that fasting can help one resist the pressure to overeat. (Of course, a doctor's visit is necessary to confirm that fasting is the right choice for you.)

But that's not to say the practice isn't without its mortal dangers, as we will see in the next chapter.

5

THE WAGES OF THIN: THE PERILS OF FASTING FOR WEIGHT LOSS

'How can anybody be too thin?'
– *The Karen Carpenter Story*, dir. Joseph Sargent (1989)

On the morning of 4 April 1921, Ellen West (1888–1921) woke feeling cheerful and hungry. Her breakfast included heaps of butter and sugar, indulgences that belied the fact that she hadn't eaten a proper meal in years. At lunch that day she left a clean plate, and she even had room enough for a dessert of coffee, chocolate creams and Easter eggs. She filled an afternoon stroll with her husband with talk of Rilke, Goethe and Tennyson. She was abidingly fond of these authors, despite having long neglected them as she remained consumed with thoughts of eating – or, more accurately, not eating. The spirit of writing carried into the evening, which she spent penning letters to friends and family. This task finished, she retired to her room.

It was the last time she would do so; she was found dead the next morning, looking, as her relations reported, 'calm and happy and peaceful'. The state suggested by her features in death had eluded her in life, and so she had taken in the night a lethal dose of poison.[1]

West's case is one of the most famous in the annals of anorexia studies. She was a patient of Ludwig Binswanger (1881–1966), the Swiss psychiatrist who pioneered existential analysis; West suffered from bulimia and anorexia nervosa for most of her adult life. She told Binswanger that her childhood was a happy one. Born into an upper-middle-class family headed by tolerant and loving parents, she grew up devouring books, studying history and writing poetry, this last pursuit adopted in service to her romantic ideals. She was headstrong, to boot. Her mother thought her a difficult child, one who defied all orders. And, by her own admission, during these early years her greatest ambition was 'to be a soldier and to die joyously with a sword in my hand'.[2] West even went so far as to claim as her own the motto *Caesar aut nihil!* ('Caesar or nothing!').[3]

As if to make good on that motto, West took a tyrannical and unyielding approach to her own body. During a trip to Sicily at age twenty, she developed an enormous appetite for the local cuisine. She gained weight, a slip from her usual fastidiousness, for which her girlfriends teased her. The raillery left her feeling humiliated – so much so that she turned to fasting and long, strenuous hikes in a bid to halt her weight gain. She succeeded more than she had expected, as her weight not only plateaued but reversed. Encouraged by her sleeker silhouette, she undertook more austerities. To friends and family, West appeared to have ended up worse for having taken the trip, the returning vacationer looking thin and haggard to them.[4]

For thirteen years after her trip to Sicily, West starved herself. The inanition affected her mood: she suffered frequent depressive episodes throughout that period. Depression led to introspection, and West offered a rationalization for her troubled relationship with food. 'My inner self is so closely connected with my body', she said, 'that the two form a unity and together constitute my "I", my unlogical, nervous, individual "I".' This persistent nervousness eclipsed all of her other interests and cast a joyless pall over the world: 'Everything is so uniform to me, so utterly indifferent,' she complained. Only her fear of food gave her purpose, spurring her to unusual practices and engendering strange thoughts. She wished fervently for 'harmless eating': that is, eating without weight gain. Because such eating was impossible, each evening she took sixty to seventy vegetable laxative tablets to purge her digestive system. What little food she ate, she later purged by vomiting. By the time she was 32, she weighed 42 kilograms (92 lb), shockingly light for any adult, but more so for West, who was reportedly tall for a woman. Indeed, she seemed little more than a skeleton. She had also ceased to menstruate.[5]

West was self-aware enough to lament how her most irrational thoughts – 'my body, my eating, my laxatives' – crowded out all others.[6] It was around this time that she began seeing Binswanger. As a result of her therapy she was able, at times, to eat normally. She even gorged herself in occasional bouts of what she called 'Fresslust', or a love of eating that verged on bestial.[7] These moments of normalcy and healthy abandon, however, were fleeting. Starvation remained an *idée fixe*; eating, a constant fantasy. West even altered her childhood dream of becoming a soldier to fit this obsession: she imagined the military life as granting, 'towards the end', consequence-free licence to eat anything she liked, 'even a big piece of Mokkatorte'.[8]

Obsession prevailed over fantasy during West's waking hours. She would eat nothing. The tension of this struggle soon grew intolerable. In fact, it drove her to several suicide attempts. She first tried by overdosing on sleeping pills. When the pills didn't work, she resorted to flinging herself bodily in what she hoped would be fatal ways – first, before a moving car and, second, out her analyst's window. West felt herself tortured by two nagging obsessions, 'hunger' and 'the dread of getting fatter', as she confided to her diary. The torture was endless. She saw 'no way out of this noose', and the realization left her with a 'horrible feeling of emptiness', one which nothing could remove.[9]

The repeated suicide attempts earned West a stay in a clinic; she was placed there by her concerned husband. Soon after her commitment, she showed signs of progress. She relaxed and seemed not as bothered by obsessive thoughts. She also ate everything placed before her: meat, potatoes, sweets, chocolate – foods she had not touched for years.[10] She wrote poetry again and read Goethe's *Faust*, a book she had once loved dearly. And she began to write the history of her own neurosis. The exercise brought her to the insight that she had let herself fall captive to a limited 'point of view', the sole focus of which was whether her actions made her 'thin or fat'.[11] Her blinkered state was such that 'all things lost their intrinsic meaning'.[12] She understood that she was enthalled to an 'uncanny power' that threatened her life.[13]

West's moments of lucidity never lasted long. Her condition again worsened, and she was transferred to another sanitarium. Here she showed little sign of improvement, becoming increasingly depressed. She made new threats of suicide. At a loss for anything more that they could do for her, her therapists diagnosed her as schizophrenic and discharged her into her husband's care. Three days later West killed herself.

Self-Starvation and Religion

Though anorexia as we know it is, historically speaking, a recent phenomenon, fatal fasts have long been a danger. And they've long posed a difficult question: when does a fast become wilful self-starvation?

The Romans were among the first to search for an answer. Documents dating from the fourth century reveal that many wealthy Roman girls were fasting to death. These girls had fallen under the influence of Christianity, a religion that exalted the spirit over the body. One such girl was Blaesilla, a noble young widow. She was the daughter of St Paula, an early Roman saint whose death from volitional starvation is likely the first fatal case of anorexia ever recorded. Blaesilla began down the same path after coming under the sway of Jerome, a priest who would himself attain sainthood. She starved herself until 'her steps tottered with weakness, her face was pale and quivering, her slender neck scarcely upheld her head.'[14] Blaesilla carried on this way for four months, her fast ending only with her death.

Many scholars of anorexia argue that such examples of fatal fasters as Blaesilla and her mother are unrelated to the disorder. Walter Vandereycken and Ron Van Deth write that 'In earlier days self-starvation as religious phenomenon or natural wonder was a meaningful figure against the background of historical periods in which the medical frame of mind played a minor or marginal role.'[15] They continue: 'Using present-day concepts for the construction of a historical bridge between fasting saints and anorexic patients looks to us like planning a transatlantic footbridge in the void.'[16] It's folly to project contemporary judgements or diagnoses on people of centuries past. What may appear as pathological behaviour today was for them simply an expression of religious fervour. This can be argued in part because the role medicine and medical knowledge played in centuries past was different in degree and kind from the role they play these days. (At any rate, no one alive today can fathom the minds of these individuals, which means, then, that judgement of their actions must be withheld.) That which can be termed anorexia as a medical condition emerged after a shift from Christendom to a secular age, with its valorization of empirical knowledge over the spiritual or mystical realms.

Anorexia in the Secular Period

As it happened, the first medicalized case of anorexia fell early in the secular turn. It came in the form of an account by British physician Richard Morton (1637–1698) published in 1689. An eighteen-year-old woman from St Mary Axe, a parish of London no longer extant, reported to Morton that her appetite 'began to Abate' in July 1684. The appetite loss continued for years, until it reduced her to something resembling 'a Skeleton only clad with Skin'. It also stopped her periods. On examination she presented with 'a coldness of the whole Body'. Like Ellen West, Morton's patient had 'a multitude of Cares and Passions of her Mind'.[17] And this restlessness persisted despite acute starvation. Indeed, never in his career had Morton seen someone so wasted.

The new wasting condition did not only affect women. A second patient to come under Morton's care was a sixteen-year-old boy. Like the young woman of St Mary Axe, the young man 'fell gradually into a total want of Appetite', an indisposition brought on by 'studying too hard and the Passions of his Mind'.[18] Morton failed to identify any single physical cause for the boy's illness, and so he laid blame on the whole 'System of Nerves', which he deemed 'distemper'd'.[19] Morton counselled his patient to abandon his studies for an idyll in the countryside, where he should breathe fresh air and drink ass's milk 'for a long time'.[20] As odd as this prescription seemed, it worked; the boy eventually recovered.

Morton was prescient in identifying such prolonged involuntary fasting as a nervous condition: today, anorexia is seen as largely a psychiatric disorder. He wasn't alone, however. Others among his contemporaries remarked on peculiar cases of inanition. Yet they put it down to a morbid state of, variously, nerves, intestines or the stomach. Not until the nineteenth century would anorexia come to be recognized as a unique disorder, thanks to an increasing number of cases coming to light. During this period, there appeared numbers of emaciated young women complaining of an inability to eat.[21] Their prevalence prompted physicians to describe the odd ailment in clinical detail.[22]

The inability to eat, they found, owed not simply to a lack of appetite. There was that, certainly, but it was attended by a host of other distinctive symptoms. Some afflicted young women reported feeling as if lumps sat in their throats and stomachs. Others behaved in a manner consistent with what would come to be called 'sitophobia', or fear of food. Still others presented with 'chorosis', a term to describe the greenish pallor many of these young women had. (Physicians today know this as hypochromic anaemia.) 'It was true that her profile was beautiful,' the narrator of English writer W. Somerset Maugham's 1915 novel *Of Human Bondage* says of the emaciated waitress Mildred Rogers; yet it was also 'as cold as marble', as well as tinged by a 'faint green' that 'gave an impression of unhealthiness'.[23] Poor health was indeed Mildred's plight – a plight shared by many women at the turn of the twentieth century who ate too little or nothing at all.

William Gull on Self-Starvation

Such indifference to food stirred physicians to hazard explanations. Many attributed it to stomach ailments of one sort or another. Two physicians, living at the same time but working separately, would posit another cause. In an 1868 address at the University of Oxford, English physician William Gull (1816–1890) advanced a novel take on self-starvation by way of the case of a seventeen-year-old woman who was 167 centimetres (5 ft 5 in.) tall and weighed a mere 37 kilograms (82 lb).[24] The young woman had grown so emaciated that she hadn't menstruated in nearly a year. She also suffered from constipation that, though mild, was chronic. She was otherwise healthy, her respiration and heart rate normal. The same could not be said, however, of her appetite. She refused all meat and dairy, and ate only scant amounts of other food. 'The condition was of simple starvation,' Gull wrote after examining her.[25] He tried various remedies, plying the girl with bichloride of mercury, syrup of iron iodine, syrup of iron phosphate and citrate of quinine. None of them worked. The cause of the problem, it seemed, was elsewhere. Even more confounding was that her appetite would return in a flash. At such moments she gorged on any food she could get, though these occasions were too rare to benefit her much.

Rare indeed was how this young woman's whole case could be described. No discomfort plagued her in her slightness, which, puzzlingly, appeared to have no physical cause. Stranger still, she had physical energy to spare. Gull described her as 'restless and active', a state belied by her wasted appearance.[26] Yet whatever the source of her abundant energy, it did not lie in the bowels; the food she did eat she digested only with difficulty. For inspiration Gull looked to Charles Chossat (he of the starved pigeon and snake animal subjects). Gull borrowed the French physiologist's approach to stimulating digestive organs with use of an India-rubber tube filled with warm water. Gull draped this medical aid along the girl's spine so that she might better absorb nutrients from the food her stomach struggled with.

Gull was left with plenty to struggle with himself. Citing the young woman's case, he stated in his Oxford address that it presented a clear example of what he termed *anorexia hysterica*. A 'morbid mental state' lay behind 'want of appetite', he claimed; disturbed individuals willed a wasted frame on themselves, the consequence of which was that no compound or elixir would cure them.[27] Called for, rather, was treatment that was 'fitted for persons of unsound mind', Gull insisted. To that end, he advised that individuals with anorexia 'be fed at regular intervals, and surrounded by persons who would have moral control over them', the latter measure disqualifying 'relations and friends', folks whom Gull deemed as being 'generally the worst attendants'.[28]

Charles Lasègue on Self-Starvation

Around the same time that Gull was investigating cases of anorexia, French physician Charles Lasègue (1816–1883) was also looking into the cause of self-starvation. The Prussian army beseiged Paris in 1870, cutting off the city's inhabitants from the means of getting food. The Parisians who were reduced to starvation proved an informative counterpoint to Lasègue's anorexia patients. The former, Lasègue noted, behaved quite differently from the latter. Long abstinence from food tended to boost rather than depress 'the aptitude for movement' in anorexia patients, he wrote.[29] Whereas a dull lassitude gripped starving Parisians – such as it had the patients of the Jewish Hospital Czyste in Warsaw – Lasègue's patients brimmed with irrepressible energy, paced nervously and fidgeted. (These days, anorexia researchers explain this restless behaviour seen in patients as due to metabolic and enzymatic changes consistent with the starvation state.)[30]

Lasègue presented his findings in a report he published in 1873, five years after Gull's Oxford address. The report detailed the unique form of self-starvation that owed, as Lasègue claimed, to 'peripheral disturbance', that is, family troubles. The French physician's diagnosis thus differed from his British counterpart's 'morbid mental state theory', despite his following Gull in naming the unusual affliction *anorexie hystérique*.[31] Notwithstanding such disagreement as to the cause, both men essentially agreed on the effect: a psychic disturbance that caused men and women to stop eating. Indeed, their descriptions of the ailment are largely the same: typically affecting young women between the ages of fifteen and twenty years; marked by interruption of the menstrual cycle (amenorrhea), constipation, restlessness and a persistent purblindness of the individuals affected as to their state; and appearing to proceed from no physical cause.[32]

Perceived Causes of Anorexia

The symptoms described by Lasègue and Gull did not escape notice by other physicians of the time. Yet there was little agreement among the latter as to the disorder's cause. Some among them identified the stomach as the sole source. Notable among this contingent were the Magenartze, a school of German and Austrian stomach specialists. The stomach was to blame for anorexia, they maintained, because it suffered a loss of sensation, which in turn meant hunger pangs – the age-old cue to take nourishment – could no longer be felt.[33]

Joining the medical men of the Magenartze in the physical-cause camp were their colleagues across the Atlantic. Physicians in the United States likewise thought anorexia had a somatic source. Neurologist William Hammond (he who offered Henry Tanner $1,000 to undertake a prolonged fast) said that anorexia proceeded from 'sensory neurosis', or exalted sensitivity, in those cases which weren't simply fraudulent. To him, food refusal represented nothing more than a perverse and wilful seeking after bodily sensation. This may sound like a psychological disorder to modern ears; but to Hammond, who disliked psychological theories, anorexia remained a problem of physiology gone awry, a disorder of the body.[34] Time would vindicate the psychological explanation, primarily because a physical cause of anorexia was nowhere to be found.

Investigating physicians did note that anorexia patients in their care shared certain tendencies: obsessions with fashion and slimness, as well as 'greater emotionality'.[35] By 1939 these traits had grown so pervasive among young people of the time that British physician John Alfred Ryle (1889–1950) predicted cases of the disorder would increase.[36]

Other physicians observed that the disorder wasn't limited to the bright young things of the interwar years; middle-class women were also susceptible to it. These women tended to be of some ambition, having earlier in life been 'stout [children] of high intelligence', very precise and attentive. Punctilious and high-minded, honest and dutiful – indeed, sometimes absurdly so – they regarded fasting as a laudable and noble practice for the self-discipline it required. Unsurprisingly, they disdained compromise and often assumed an authoritative attitude. They could also, at times, be reserved and unsociable, taking into their confidence, at most, one or two friends.[37]

Though most individuals with anorexia were women, the disorder was not without its male victims, perhaps the most notable among the latter being Franz Kafka (1883–1924). Lonely, depressive and a perfectionist, the twentieth-century Czech writer ticked several diagnostic boxes. Like Ellen West, he would fast as he watched family and friends dine. Also like West, Kafka fantasized about gorging himself. To keep these unwelcome imaginings at bay, he ran, swam and did gymnastics, taking to these activities with compulsive fervour. Kafka got his desired result. 'I am the thinnest human being I know', he wrote.[38] He seemed well pleased with this distinction.

Alarming thinness was a pleasing distinction to an American contemporary of Kafka's. Standing 183 centimetres (6 ft) in height, horror fiction writer H. P. Lovecraft (1890–1937) never permitted his weight to exceed 66 kilograms (146 lb). He deliberately underate and at times fasted, all so he might retain his preternaturally slim physique. The strict weight management reduced Lovecraft to a walking cadaver to onlookers. 'Folds of skin hanging from a skeleton' was how a friend described him. This friend went on to note that Lovecraft's eyes were 'sunk in sockets like burnt holes in a blanket' and his 'artist's hands and fingers nothing but claws'. Really, the friend concluded, the 'man was dead except for his nerves'.[39] However disturbing the sight of Lovecraft was to others, to Lovecraft himself it was a delight. He regarded it as the mark of a thorough gentleman.

Ellen West, Franz Kafka and H. P. Lovecraft alike fell captive to an impossible ideal that curdled a healthy impulse to manage caloric intake into a chronic illness. The three figures

shared circumstances of relative privilege and a will sur-
passed in strength only by a creative impulse. These factors
appear to support a psychological explanation for anorexia.
Present-day medical professionals maintain that certain
biological and cultural factors also contribute to the disorder.
Trouble with family members may lead an individual to
become anorexic, as may hormonal imbalances or exposure
at an early age to media representations of physical ideals.
The difference between a strict yet physically harmless diet
and a dangerous illness may be any one of several hidden
vulnerabilities. Thus the greatest danger that attends fasting
is perhaps the possibility of triggering a latent propensity to
anorexia or some other eating disorder. 'People can go on a
fast and think that it is going to be healthy for them, and it
may in fact be,' notes Sondra Kronberg, a nutrition therapist
and the founder of the Eating Disorder Collaborative, 'but
then they'll come off and they'll binge for weeks.'[40] Studies
have shown that fasting is correlated with a higher incidence
of bulimia.[41] Even fasts of short duration carry risks.
'Intermittent fasting is a gateway to an eating disorder,'
says registered dietitian Evelyn Tribole.[42]

Forewarned is forearmed. Those wanting to fast for weight
loss should consult their physician before doing so. Really,
consultation with a physician is essential even when the
diet undertaken seems to have won popular approval. The
most acclaimed diet can encourage dangerous behaviour
in the name of health and well-being, as a few unfortunate
American bohemians discovered in the mid-1960s.

George Ohsawa's Macrobiotic Diet

In 1965, Sakurazawa Nyoiti (1893–1966), who came to be known by his pen name, George Ohsawa, published *You Are All Sanpaku*. The Japanese physician's slim volume details how most people in the West – such as Richard Nixon and Brigitte Bardot, to name two – suffer from a condition of *sanpaku*, Japanese for 'three whites'. The whites in question are the portions of the sclera visible between an individual's iris and eyelids. Two visible portions suggest a state of sound health; three, impending misfortune and growing inward corruption.

Ohsawa's medical theory found purchase with a rather specific crowd. It consisted, as one contemporary newspaper account explained, of individuals who were 'smooth faced with short hair'. All middle-class men and women, they were 'ex-drug users' with 'candid' and 'slightly righteous' personalities, the article went on. They were similar still in that all were 'somewhat lonely', not to mention 'more than a little disenchanted with contemporary American life'.[43] No more ideal a coterie could be imagined for the diet devised by Ohsawa, who promised it would clear up *sanpaku*. It caught countercultural fire as sundry beatniks and nonconformists forswore aubergine, tomato, potato, sugar, soft drinks, coffee, fruit (both its flesh and juice), desserts and meat.

Ohsawa's dietetics carried adherents through several stages, or 'regimens'. The early regimens offered a relatively varied menu of vegetables, fish and grains. The later regimens offered grains alone, culminating in 'Regimen Number 7', which consisted solely of brown rice.[44] Only the most disciplined of the dieters under Ohsawa's direction managed to reach this last stage. Ohsawa also forbade his adherents to drink anything more than meagre amounts of water on the basis that too much of the stuff damaged kidneys. (Whether adherents were drinking too much water could be told by the colour of their urine: fluid even one shade lighter than a cup of English Breakfast tea meant they needed to ease off.) Ohsawa's regimens might seem insanely limited to most sensible people, yet they presented 'the easiest, simplest, and wisest' diet of all – if its creator was to be believed.[45] Regimen Number 7 arrived as a panacea. It purported to prevent apoplexy, halt appendicitis, remedy stomach aches and reverse sterility. To women it held out a special attraction, promising to save them from what Ohsawa described as 'a tragedy more cataclysmic than thermonuclear destructions' – the continued growth of leg hair.[46] These varied benefits supplied incentive enough for sticking to the plan.

Whether as deliverance from health disaster or simply the personal apocalypse of hairy legs, Ohsawa's regimens struck early adopters as nothing short of miraculous. Even dieters who did not progress beyond the least restrictive early regimens reported happy effects. William Dufty (1916–2002), a journalist who penned the introduction to the definitive English translation of You Are All Sanpaku, claimed that the diet stripped him of nearly 14 kilograms (30 lb). What's more, it shrank his hemorrhoids, banished his chronic headaches, pinkened anew his pyorrhea-plagued gums and dried his excessive perspiration – all afflictions that had dogged Dufty through a lifetime. So thorough was his transformation from the diet that Dufty came to regard the diet's creator as something of a Pygmalion and himself 'as an Oshawa mannequin'.[47] Buoyed by greater health and well-being, Dufty became a fixture at the Ohsawa Foundation, which distributed special macrobiotic foodstuffs; he became an evangelist, if a reluctant one, for the diet itself. 'Overweight friends of both sexes drove me berserk asking for the secret,' he wrote, the pestering becoming so constant, in fact, that he 'grew weary of explaining' the 'regimen to get healthy' that he had adopted.[48]

As Dufty watched his weight drop and his health improve, he found little reason to attempt the strictest of Ohsawa's regimens. Rather he contented himself with the most liberal of them, which consisted of brown rice, vegetables and fish. Some time spent in prison, however, disrupted his diet. He was offered little beyond potato salad and canned meat. Dufty, at this point still Ohsawa's mannequin, turned his nose up at these. His only recourse, then, was to fast. Nervous at first about going without food, he looked to fellow devotees of Ohsawa's regimens for encouragement. No less than his adviser at the Ohsawa Foundation told him that as someone who had been 'macrobiotic for almost four months', he was well positioned to go 'without food for thirty days at least with no danger at all'. The worst effect was that he'd 'get a little thin', but the total effect would be thoroughly beneficial. As the adviser told Dufty, 'if there's anything wrong with you there's nothing like a good fast.'[49]

It happened that Dufty never found the chance to put his fasting endurance to the test; he was released from custody after six days. The claim that Ohsawa's macrobiotic regimens put dieters in a strong position for enduring a long fast, however, did get put to the test. Another of Ohsawa's followers, Beth Ann Simon, undertook Regimen Number 7 in February 1965. The free-spirited 24-year-old resident of New York's bohemian Greenwich Village ate nothing but brown rice dusted with gomasio, a Japanese seasoning of salt, dried seaweed and sesame seeds. She took this meal three times daily and washed it down with the merest sips of water. Simon's friends and family became alarmed when they learned the extent of her diet. They begged her to eat more. Simon refused. She likewise refused to see a doctor after Regimen Number 7 left her bedridden. Egging Simon on in her defiance was none other than Ohsawa himself. In a letter to his follower, he opined that she was 'one of the luckiest people in the world' for her dogged adherence to the programme to which she had been granted access: 'Stay on Diet 7 and you will get well,' he promised.[50]

Whatever wellness lay in store for Simon would not find her in this earthly realm. She stuck with the most extreme form of the diet for three more days after she received the letter from Ohsawa. In November 1965 Simon died on her diet's fourth day, her mortal remains weighing a mere 32 kilograms (70 lb).

Simon's death came just as Ohsawa's macrobiotic diet was finding wider popularity. The trend prompted intervention from the *Journal of the American Medical Association Council on Foods and Nutrition*. In 1971, the publication warned that 'the concepts proposed in Zen constitute a major public health problem, and are dangerous to its adherents.'[51] (Ohsawa linked his diet to Zen Buddhism, despite disavowals by that faith's authorities.) It went on to detail the medical problems such a diet can cause, including scurvy, protein deficiency (hypoproteinia), low calcium (hypocalcemia), loss of kidney function, emaciation and other forms of malnutrition.[52] The *Journal*'s warning fell on many ears that had been deafened by the promise of glowing health and longevity. Yet for all the nibbling of vegetables and brown rice, in actuality the reward for the diet's followers was only serious nutritional deficiencies.

The Dangers of Fasting Diets

As fasting diets go, Ohsawa's Zen macrobiotic regimens are among the most notoriously extreme. Yet fasting diets need not be so drastic to present health dangers. Even relatively brief fasts harbour risks. The starvation diets of the 1960s, which were discussed in an earlier chapter, can aggravate gout, heart problems and other ailments. Diabetics are especially vulnerable to fasting diets. Muslims with hypoglycaemia who fast during Ramadan, for example, may aggravate their condition, particularly if they continue insulin treatment through the holy month.[53]

In fact, fasting diets can kill even the heartiest folks. Completely healthy student athletes have suffered dangerous side effects from crash-fasts to lose weight quickly. In 1997, for example, three healthy collegiate wrestlers died after fasting to qualify for competition.[54] In 1927 the *Auckland Star* reported on an otherwise healthy 43-year-old lieutenant-colonel who took to subsisting on little more than fruits, vegetables and grains. For breakfast, he ate two grapes and an orange. His lunch consisted of a potato and three raw cabbage leaves, a spoonful each of grated carrot and beet, two dry biscuits and some butter. He ate no dinner. After following this diet for some time, he died of heart failure. His cause of death was determined to be starvation owing to a 'peculiar and distorted view', as the *Star* article put it.[55]

Dinner Time

Such unfortunate incidents show that, even without a pre-disposition to anorexia or other eating disorders, individuals may suffer ill effects from fasting diets. And these effects can extend to their larger social sphere. Fasting is a solitary activity; as such, it can isolate people, severing them from the customs and traditions shared by family and friends. Chief among these customs are mealtimes.

Dinner, for example, is often taken for granted; it's an event that happens nearly every night – and seemingly has for generations – a cosy constant reaching into the dim past. To believe this about dinner, however, is to cherish a mis-conception: as most middle-class people enjoy it, the nightly ritual of nourishment evolved rather recently, historically speaking. Prior to the eighteenth century, most families of modest income dined in silence; the main meal of the day carried little significance, and thus neither did the behaviour of those observing it. It was only with the Enlightenment and greater prosperity that a new conception was developed as to how family and friends should behave towards one another, as well as of the pleasure to be had from domesticity. Dining with loved ones was now meant to be pleasurable, an occasion for mutual sympathy, friendship and affection.[56]

'I allowed . . . an hour for dinner,' wrote Oliver Goldsmith in the *Vicar of Wakefield* (1766), 'which time was taken up in innocent mirth between my wife and daughters, and in philosophical arguments between my son and me.'[57]

Such prandial conviviality took on greater importance for bourgeois families living in the tumultuous cities of Europe and the United States. In these metropolises people of different professions, cultures and class backgrounds mingled indiscriminately. Starting in the eighteenth century, the dinner table became a haven from the social tumult outside, a place to reaffirm shared values – be they philosophical, religious or otherwise – and one's place in the world.[58] The Enlightenment brought a shift in social structures and, for many, time that might previously have been spent with family came to be spent at work and engaged in outside interests and relationships. As such, dining together became even more precious.[59]

The highly valued dinner together endures to this day throughout Europe and the United States. (This is not to suggest that dinner lacks similar esteem in the rest of the world, only to suggest that its value may rest on reasons quite different from those which prevail in the West.) Marketing specialist Clotaire Rapaille conducted a number of surveys and found that Americans still associate dinner with domestic pleasure. 'When we think about home,' he writes, 'one of the first images to come to mind usually involves a big family meal.'[60] Indeed, one survey participant stated that she 'looked forward to dinner every night' with her parents and two brothers.[61] At these gatherings together they discussed 'the day's events and upcoming plans for the following day'.[62] She went on to characterize the dinner scene as 'a warm environment, full of love and nurturing'.[63] Interestingly, dinner loses nothing of its charm when circumstances prevent it from being taken regularly; meals shared at holidays – Christmas, Easter and, in the United States, Thanksgiving – assume all the importance to families of meals taken together nightly.

The emotional significance of communal meals makes the very idea of forsaking them – for a better figure! – seem a dismal gesture of lonely egoism. Such rejection entails reducing conviviality, gastronomy and pleasure to a matter of mere nutrition, of calories, minerals and vitamins. Eating together, on the other hand, turns 'the exclusive selfishness of eating' into 'a habit of being gathered together such as is seldom attainable on occasions of a higher and intellectual order', wrote the early twentieth-century German sociologist Georg Simmel.[64] Perhaps this is why it is more often the affluent who fast willingly; the poor are far less likely to refuse a generous meal eaten in safety and comfort among friends and family. For who can say when that opportunity might be denied them?

Fasting around the Family Dinner

Happily, you can fast and have your dinner, too. To begin with, most total fasts are of short duration, lasting between two and three days. And intermittent fasts give one a choice as to which meal to skip. Dinner has become an occasion of deep meaning; one should therefore skip the meal with the least emotional content. 'In virtually all societies', writes nutrition scholar Elaine McIntosh, 'the meal with the least emotional weight is the first meal of the day (breakfast).'[65] Breakfast is also the meal least likely to be eaten with family members. Of all the varieties of fasting and dieting plans we've thus far encountered, Edward Dewey's No-Breakfast Plan seems like the most agreeable to both a dieter and their friends and family.

Since the publication of Dewey's plan, science has confirmed what he intuited: so long as you limit eating to an eight-hour window (from, say, 7:00 a.m. to 3.00 p.m.), you can experience health benefits and weight loss. And though those same studies state that skipping dinner lends the most rewards, people who opted to skip breakfast found that they too lost weight and felt healthier.[66] Even more promising, the breakfast-skippers did not try to make up for the calories lost at breakfast by eating a larger lunch.[67]

And so, with this last danger averted, we can turn our sights to the future of fasting.

EPILOGUE: OF APPS AND APPETITE – THE FUTURE OF FASTING

'When the stomach is full, it is easy to talk of fasting.'
– St Jerome

As I hope the pages you've read to this point have amply shown, I know much more today about the virtues and challenges of fasting than I did in those days of watching my grandfather forgo schnitzel in abstinence. It's clear to me now that he simply partook of a long tradition of questing after health and equanimity.

Despite my own failed first foray into fasting, I'm happy to say that I have since met with success. I now practise a form of 16:8 fasting, in which I confine my daily eating to two meals taken within an eight-hour window. Except for infrequent occasions when I would risk being discourteous, I go without dinner. I've been at it for nearly two years as I write this in 2022. The lifestyle overhaul called for by this kind of regimen was surprisingly easy for me; rarely do I feel any hunger pangs in the evening. And the benefits have been many. Well-being suffuses me. My vigour has gone undiminished, has perhaps even grown. My weight essentially controls itself. My blood pressure and heart rate are at healthy levels. Plus – and I can't emphasize enough what an unexpected boon this has proven – I have a portion of my life back. How wonderful it is not to face having to make (or order in) dinner, eat and do dishes after a long day at work. My evenings have become my own. I can read, sketch, write, sew or do anything else I like.

This is all to say that the question 'Why fast?' is one that I have answered for myself. And the practice seems quite effortless now that I've grown used to it.

Yet if I needed help in skipping meals, there's more assistance than ever before now available. Flagging willpower? There's an app for that. A few, in fact. One called MyFast promises to help you 'soothe your way to your fasting intervals', and it includes 'a progress bar' that demonstrates how far along you're from reaching your goal.[1] Another, BodyFast, lets you choose a weekly fasting plan. You can also receive individual plans formulated by one of the app's coaches.

Custom fasts aren't limited to apps. Increasingly more regimens are being developed to account for an individual's unique physiology. Just as dieting has become more personalized, so too has fasting. The Toronto Metabolic Clinic, for example, offers fasting programmes calibrated for each patient to cure everything from type 2 diabetes to polycystic ovary syndrome.

This personalized approach to fasting is part of the larger vogue for 'biohacking', or the means by which an individual works around the limitations of the human body to access untapped abilities and potential. Geoffrey Woo (b. 1988), CEO of the Silicon Valley nootropics company H.V.M.N., is one such eager biohacker. In addition to running his company, Woo, who himself fasts for 44 to 48 weeks a year, oversees a thriving Facebook and Slack community of more than 6,000 members devoted to the practice.[2] Called WeFast, the community shares tips – new fasters should remember to consume electrolytes, for example – as well as encouragement and fellowship. 'I joined to have possibly find [sic] a friend to fast with,' reads one testimonial from a newbie. 'I'm currently on my first fast and am hitting 70 hours.'[3] WeFast members in San Francisco meet at a local café every Wednesday to break their fasts, which for some run as long as 36 hours, over eggs and smoked salmon. And for shining examples many of them need look no further than the C-suites where they work. 'I'm inspired by the fasting of Jack Dorsey and other Silicon Valley entrepreneurs,' writes another new member. 'My ultimate goal is to lose weight, increase productivity, and improve my health.'[4]

For these newbie fasters there are a seemingly infinite variety of options. The Snake Diet has fasters drink a saline solution to keep hunger pangs at bay. With the 16:8 method, all daily eating must be done in an eight- to ten-hour window. And a 24-hour fast once or twice a week defines the Eat–Stop–Eat diet. If none of these more arithmetically regimented plans suits you, the Warrior Diet lets you fast by day and feast by night. And for the most improvisational among the fasting-curious, there's Spontaneous Meal Skipping, which recommends that you fast simply when you feel like it. Even people who quail at the idea of going without food altogether for any amount of time have recourse to calorie-restricted diets that claim to mimic fasting's effects. Add to all these Calorie Cycling (restriction of caloric intake to every other day), the 5:2 diet (confining intake to 600 calories two days per week), time-restricted eating (eating during a twelve- or eighteen-hour window) and the ProLon fast (a five-day diet that limits you to 500 calories each day), and you realize that the contemporary moment offers a veritable smorgasbord of novel fasts.

How to choose among them? Those who cannot find a community with whom to compare fasting diets in physical meet-ups may swap tips and commiserate in fasting forums and Internet communities. Unlike the hunger artists of yore, who had to travel from city to city, fasters now come right to your home, courtesy of YouTube. Their videos documenting their fasts allow you to experience the practice vicariously. A British couple whose YouTube handle is 'Have Butter Will Travel' share the trials and tribulations of a five-day fast. They end the first day looking tired and haggard yet also confident that they can continue, buoyed by water sprinkled with pink salt and by sips of bone broth.[5] An American woman documents her three-day juice cleanse. Her video shows her drinking six specially made juices a day, at a daily cost of about \$34.50. On the first day, she reports feeling famished and bloated. By the second day she is 'feeling good', but confesses she is still struggling with hunger pangs. The third day sees her losing the ability to focus on work and feeling lethargic, only to end the day feeling energetic. Overall, she says she enjoyed the experience and promises to update viewers with any lasting effects.[6]

For more traditional fasters, there are still spas and retreats. The Kloster Pernegg fasting clinic in Austria attracts visitors from across Europe. Housed in a former monastery, it brings a contemplative atmosphere to the practice. 'Many of the people there are there not to lose weight,' my father, who's a frequent visitor, told me, 'but to achieve a sense of clarity and health.'[7] While sipping herbal broths and juices, visitors spend their day hiking, sunbathing and meditating. For them, fasting is a secular spiritual practice, one in which communion with the self has replaced communion with the divine. At Sura Detox in Berrynarbor, England, fasters can choose either a juice or water fast, as well as engage in a number of stimulating activities. Tai-chi, meditation and yoga sessions, counselling sessions, nutritional talks and food prep sessions are all available to help beguile the time while fasting. Sura Detox aims not only to improve your health, but to deepen your 'understanding about your relationship to food, each other, and your life's choices'.[8]

Fasting has become more social. Gone are the days when hunger artists starved alone; now they can tap into any number of forums to commiserate with their fellow fasters. Is this an unqualified good? That depends on the goals of the fast. For those seeking to lose weight through fasting yet unable to afford a pricey stay at a fasting clinic, virtual communities can provide much-needed support. Dieters who belong to virtual communities have been shown to adhere to their goals more consistently. It follows, then, that fasters would experience similar benefits.[9]

Apps can also provide support, and they too have been shown to promote weight loss and physical activity.[10] Users claim apps help keep them on track by encouraging them to record their progress. If an app includes a human coaching component, then users report even more success.[11] And some apps make losing weight or fasting into a game, urging users to rack up points or compete against other users, all of which appears to heighten motivation in certain individuals.

But for those who want to use a fast to change habits, both of mind and body, social media and apps can only prove a distraction, prompting one to focus on the app or community and not on one's body and state of mind. Indeed, they turn fasting into yet another occasion to interact even more with the devices that already dominate our lives. How could you gain a different view on your life under such circumstances? As we saw in the first chapter, we live in an increasingly obesogenic environment: that is, an environment conducive to habitual overeating. Fasting can break this habit, whether through skipping breakfast or going without food for an entire week. In both cases, individuals seek to develop a more nuanced relationship with their body and its needs. In this new state of mind, they may be able to imagine other ways of avoiding overconsumption: walking or cycling rather than driving, for example, or forgoing the latest fashions. A mindful fast can open the doors to other practices that are healthier for humans and the environment they live in.

As consoling as apps and virtual communities may be, they are still a form of consumption. If the goal of a fast is to consume less in general, then they can only undermine that purpose. In the end, however, fasting's future is its present and its past. It's simply a matter of not eating. And this is why – no matter how many apps you have or how many communities you join – fasting comes down to one thing: willpower. This has been the challenge that would-be fasters have faced for millennia. Today's obesogenic environment, with its ever-proliferating temptations, makes the act of not eating even more difficult. Nonetheless, I hope your willpower has been bolstered by this account of the compelling history and science of fasting. Despite its difficulty, fasting, when done in moderation and under the care of a trained professional, can deliver health benefits that make avoiding temptation well worth the effort.

REFERENCES

1 A HUNGER FOR MORE: FASTING AND ITS PURPOSES FROM ANTIQUITY TO THE PRESENT

1 Quoted in Adam Gopnik, 'Can We Live Longer but Stay Younger?', *New Yorker*, www.newyorker.com, 13 May 2019.

2 C. Miller and K. H. Coble, 'Cheap Food Policy: Fact or Rhetoric?', *Food Policy*, XXXII/1 (2007), pp. 98–111.

3 C. A. Monteiro et al., 'NOVA: The Star Shines Bright', *World Nutrition*, VII/1–3 (2016), p. 30.

4 C. A. Monteiro et al., 'Ultra-Processed Products Are Becoming Dominant in the Global Food System', *Obesity Reviews: An Official Journal of the International Association for the Study of Obesity*, XIV (2013), p. 23.

5 Brian Wansink, *Mindless Eating: Why We Eat More Than We Think* (New York, 2006), pp. 1–2.

6 L. Jahns, A. M. Siega-Riz and B. M. Popkin, 'The Increasing Prevalence of Snacking among U.S. Children from 1977 to 1996', *Journal of Pediatrics*, CXXXVIII/4 (2001), p. 495.

7 Eliana Zeballos, Jessica E. Todd and Brandon Restrepo. 'Frequency and Time of Day That Americans Eat: A Comparison of Data from the American Time Use Survey and the National Health and Nutrition Examination Survey', *Economic Research Service Technical Bulletin* (2019), p. 7.

8 M. N. Laska et al., 'Situational Characteristics of Young Adults' Eating Occasions: A Real-Time Data Collection Using Personal Digital Assistants', *Public Health Nutrition*, XIV/3 (2011), p. 2.

9 The effect of television watching, music listening and intellectual work on eating comes from J.-P. Chaput et al., 'Modern Sedentary Activities Promote Overconsumption of Food

in Our Current Obesogenic Environment', *Obesity Reviews*, XII/5 (2011), p. 12.

10 Paavo O. Airola, *How to Keep Slim, Healthy, and Young with Juice Fasting* (Phoenix, AZ, 1971), p. 16.

11 John Ciardi, *How Does a Poem Mean?* (Boston, MA, 1959), p. 765.

12 Ibid.

13 Jules Blumensohn, 'The Fast among North American Indians', *American Anthropologist*, XXXV/3 (1933), pp. 454–5.

14 Ibid., p. 453.

15 Ibid.

16 Ibid.

17 Ibid.

18 Caroline Westbrook, 'Why Do Muslims Fast for Ramadan and What Does It Represent?', *Metro*, www.metro.co.uk, 25 April 2021.

19 Civil Service of India, 'Hindu Fasting in the Workplace: An Awareness Guide for Staff and Managers' (15 October 2019), pp. 3–4.

20 Quoted in Ajahn Brahmavamso, 'The Time and Place for Eating', www.urbandharma.org, 22 June 2002.

21 Andrew Jotischky, *A Hermit's Cookbook: Monks, Food and Fasting in the Middle Ages* (London, 2011), p. 28.

22 Maurice E. Shils and Moshe Shike, *Modern Nutrition in Health and Disease*, 10th edn (Philadelphia, PA, 2006), p. 10.

23 John R. Butterly and Jack Shepherd, *Hunger: The Biology and Politics of Starvation* (Hanover, NH, 2010), pp. 60–62.

24 Ibid., pp. 66–7.

25 Ibid., p. 92.

26 Ibid.

27 Christopher D. Saudek and Philip Felig, 'The Metabolic Events of Starvation', *American Journal of Medicine*, LX/1 (1976), p. 117.

28 Ancel Keys, *The Biology of Human Starvation* (Minneapolis, MN, 1950), p. 3.

29 F. R. de Azevedo, Dimas Ikeoka and Bruno Caramelli, 'Effects of Intermittent Fasting on Metabolism in Men', *Revista Da Associação Médica Brasileira*, English edn, LIX/59.2 (2013), p. 168.

30 William Cronon, *Changes in the Land: Indians, Colonists, and the Ecology of New England* (New York, 2013), p. 71.

31 Ibid.

32 Leo Pruimboom et al., 'Influence of a 10-Day Mimic of Our Ancient Lifestyle on Anthropometrics and Parameters of Metabolism and Inflammation: The "Study of Origin"', *Biomed Research International* (2016), pp. 1–7.

33 Jean-Hervé Lignot and Yvon LeMaho, 'A History of Modern Research into Fasting, Starvation, and Inanition', in *Comparative Physiology of Fasting, Starvation, and Food Limitation*, ed. Marshall D. McCue (Berlin, 2012), p. 14.

34 Ibid.

35 Tobias Wang, Carrie C. Y. Hung and David J. Randall, 'The Comparative Physiology of Food Deprivation: From Feast to Famine', *Annual Review of Physiology*, LXVIII/1 (2006), p. 231.

36 René Groscolas and Jean-Patrice Robin, 'Long-Term Fasting and Re-Feeding in Penguins', *Comparative Biochemistry and Physiology Part A: Molecular and Integrative Physiology*, CXXVIII/3 (2001), p. 646.

37 Ibid., p. 649. The emperor penguin's mate usually returns in time to relieve him of his hungry vigil. If she doesn't, the male must leave his egg to march some 200 kilometres over sea ice to open water, a trek which costs him 20 kilograms of additional muscle mass. Not to make the journey costs him his life.

38 Jeremy Hance, 'The World's Best Mother: Meet the Octopus That Guards Its Eggs for Over Four Years', *Monga Bay*, www.news. mongabay.com, 30 July 2014.

2 FOOD FOR THOUGHT: FASTING THROUGH THE AGES

1 Knut Hamsun, *Hunger* (New York, 1920), p. 88.

2 'After 44 Days, David Blaine's out of His Box', *The Scotsman*, www.scotsman.com, 20 October 2003.

3 'Interview with David Blaine', *Larry King Live*, CNN, transcripts. cnn.com, 5 November 2003.

4 George Rosen, 'Metabolism: The Evolution of a Concept', in *Essays on History of Nutrition and Dietetics*, ed. Adelia M. Beeuwkes, E. Neige Todhunter and Emma Seifrit Weigley (Chicago, IL, 1967), p. 60.

5 Paul Studtmann, 'Living Capacities and Vital Heat in Aristotle', *Ancient Philosophy*, XXIV/2 (2004), pp. 367–9.

6 Ibid., p. 368.

7 Erasistratus was also noteworthy for collecting the largest
   medical fee on record.
8 Quoted in Graham Lusk, *Nutrition* (New York, 1964),
   p. 12.
9 Ibid.
10 Ibid.
11 *The Encyclopaedia Britannica Guide to the 100 Most Influential
   Scientists: The Most Important Scientists from Ancient Greece
   to the Present Day* (London, 2008), p. 48.
12 Ibid.
13 Quoted in J. M. Stillman and Sherwood J. B. Sugden, 'Paracelsus
   as a Reformer in Medicine', *Monist*, XXIX/4 (1919), p. 532.
14 Ibid.
15 Ibid., p. 531.
16 Ibid.
17 Ibid., p. 542.
18 Lusk, *Nutrition*, p. 29.
19 Quoted in Teresa Hollerbach, 'The Weighing Chair of Sanctorius
   Sanctorius: A Replica', *NTM*, XXVI (2018), p. 124.
20 Ibid., p. 121.
21 E. Neige Todhunter, 'Development of Knowledge in Nutrition',
   in *Essays on History of Nutrition and Dietetics*, ed. Beeuwkes,
   Todhunter and Weigley, pp. 48–9.
22 Elmer Verner McCollum, *A History of Nutrition: The Sequence
   of Ideas in Nutrition Investigations* (Boston, MA, 1957), pp. 187–8.
   As McCollum notes, amateur investigators could boast of royalty
   in their ranks. England's King Charles II became occupied with
   his own form. He 'had the curiosity of weighing himself very
   frequently', said the natural philosopher Sir Robert Moray of
   the monarch, doing so after eating, sleeping and 'riding abroad'.
   A game of tennis led to a loss of nearly 1 kg, which 'two draughts
   of liquor after play' restored, the sovereign noted of himself.
   Dinner, meanwhile, tended to end in double the weight gain
   brought on by post-game tipples.
23 Quoted in Lusk, *Nutrition*, p. 66.
24 Ibid., p. 67.
25 Ibid.
26 A tax farmer in pre-revolutionary France was usually a connected individual who collected taxes from the people on behalf

of the Crown in exchange for a bonus, which came as a portion of the taxes collected.

27 Todhunter, 'Development of Knowledge in Nutrition', p. 42.
28 Richard L. Kremer, *The Thermodynamics of Life and Experimental Physiology, 1770–1880* (New York, 1990), pp. 65–8.
29 Todhunter, 'Development of Knowledge in Nutrition', p. 49.
30 Quoted in Lusk, *Nutrition*, p. 63.
31 Kremer, *Thermodynamics of Life*, pp. 82–3.
32 McCollum, *History of Nutrition*, pp. 64–5.
33 Spallanzani's experiment resembled one conducted about a century before. In the earlier experiment, the French polymath René Antoine Ferchault de Réaumur used metal tubes rather than linen sacks, and he used only kites and dogs as his animal subjects.
34 McCollum, *History of Nutrition*, pp. 65–6.
35 Kremer, *Thermodynamics of Life*, p. 113.
36 Ibid., pp. 113–16.
37 Ibid., p. 115.
38 'Dr Chossat on Inanition', *Edinburgh Medical and Surgical Journal*, LXI/158 (1844), pp. 156–8.
39 Ibid., p. 161.
40 Ibid.
41 Ibid., pp. 159–60.
42 Ibid., p. 162.
43 Ibid.
44 Liebig's hope may have owed in part to childhood memories of 1814, the famous 'Year Without a Summer' in which an erupting volcano threw so much soot and ash into the atmosphere that it brought on months of abnormal cold. Agriculture was dealt a grievous blow, and the resulting crop failures led to rampant hunger.
45 It should be noted that Englishman William Prout preceded Liebig in identifying these three nutrients.
46 Rosen, 'Metabolism', p. 63.
47 Quoted in Ancel Keys, *The Biology of Human Starvation* (Minneapolis, MN, 1950), p. 784.
48 Richard Baron Howard, *An Inquiry into the Morbid Effects of Deficiency of Food* (London, 1839), p. 19.
49 Ibid.

50 Ibid., p. 20.

51 Ibid., p. 27.

52 Keys, *Biology of Human Starvation*, pp. 810–13.

53 Quoted ibid., p. 810.

54 Quoted ibid., p. 812.

55 Quoted ibid.

56 Augustí Nieto-Galan, 'Useful Charlatans: Giovanni Succi and Stefano Merlatti's Fasting Contest in Paris, 1886', *Science in Context*, XXXIII/4 (2020), pp. 405–22.

57 Francis Gano Benedict et al., *A Study of Prolonged Fasting* (Washington, DC, 1915), p. 23.

58 Ibid., p. 24.

59 Ibid., p. 27.

60 Ibid.

61 Ibid., p. 36.

62 Ibid., p. 67.

63 Ibid., p. 157.

64 Ibid., p. 187.

65 Ibid., pp. 182–5.

66 Ibid., p. 190.

67 Keys, *Biology of Human Starvation*, p. 779. Levanzin began fasting three days after his arrival in Boston, and he did not have time to become familiar enough with the mental acuity tests he was to perform under starvation conditions.

68 Howard D. Marsh, 'Individual and Sex Differences Brought out by Fasting', *Psychological Review*, XXIII/6 (1916), p. 445.

69 John A. Glaze, 'Sensitivity to Odors and Other Phenomena During a Fast', *American Journal of Psychology*, XL/4 (1928), p. 575.

70 Graham Lusk, *The Elements of the Science of Nutrition* (Philadelphia, PA, 1906), p. 54.

71 Quoted in Keys, *Biology of Human Starvation*, p. 35.

72 Benedict did make some small changes. He disallowed his subjects any butter, but he let them have apple jelly instead. And he allowed them extra portions of spinach and other bulky foods.

73 Keys, *Biology of Human Starvation*, pp. 34–62.

74 Myron Winick, *Hunger Disease: Studies by the Jewish Physicians in the Warsaw Ghetto* (New York, 1979), p. xi.

75 Quoted ibid., p. 15.

76 Ibid.
77 Ibid., pp. 16–18.
78 Quoted ibid., p. 43.
79 Quoted ibid., p. 5.
80 Ibid., p. ix.
81 Keys, *Biology of Human Starvation*, pp. 835–7.
82 Ibid., p. 837.
83 Sharman Apt Russell, *Hunger: An Unnatural History* (New York, 2006), p. 126.
84 Todd Tucker, *The Great Starvation Experiment: The Heroic Men Who Starved So That Millions Could Live* (New York, 2006), p. 99.
85 Keys, *Biology of Human Starvation*, p. 895.
86 Ibid., p. 903.
87 Ibid., p. 76.
88 Russell, *Unnatural History*, p. 134.
89 Indeed, those not receiving extra protein recovered their strength faster.
90 Russell, *Unnatural History*, p. 133.
91 One man ensured that he always had a chocolate bar or two at hand.
92 Keys, *Biology of Human Starvation*, p. 843.
93 Ibid., p. 847.
94 Ibid., p. 843.
95 Ibid.
96 Ibid., p. 1054.
97 Ibid.
98 Ibid., p. 1056.
99 Ibid., p. 1046.
100 Ibid.
101 Ibid.
102 Ibid., p. 617.

3 THE PHYSICIAN WITHIN: FASTING FOR HEALTH

1 Mark Twain, 'My Debut as a Literary Person' [1903], https://americanliterature.com, accessed 11 August 2022.
2 Jeanette Winterson, 'Why I Checked into a Fasting Clinic', *The Telegraph*, www.telegraph.co.uk, 14 April 2017.

3 Ibid.

4 Ibid.

5 Ian Belcher, 'The Enema Within', *The Guardian*, www.theguardian.com, 9 March 2002.

6 Judith Thurman, 'The Fast Lane', *New Yorker*, 3 September 2007, www.newyorker.com, accessed 2 August 2022.

7 Arlene Harris, 'All or Nothing: The People Who Are Intermittent Fasting Their Way to Weight-Loss', *The Independent*, www.independent.ie, 11 September 2019.

8 M. Mattson and Ruiqian Wan, 'Beneficial Effects of Intermittent Fasting and Caloric Restriction on the Cardiovascular and Cerebrovascular Systems', *Journal of Nutritional Biochemistry*, XVI/3 (2005), p. 130.

9 Ibid.

10 M. Remely et al., 'Increased Gut Microbiota Diversity and Abundance of *Faecalibacterium Prausnitzii* and *Akkermansia* after Fasting: A Pilot Study', *Wien Klinische Wochenschrift*, 127 (2015), p. 394.

11 Mattson and Wan, 'Beneficial Effects of Intermittent Fasting', p. 135.

12 Ruth E. Patterson and Dorothy D. Sears, 'Metabolic Effects of Intermittent Fasting', *Annual Review of Nutrition*, 37 (2017), pp. 380–81.

13 Ibid., p. 381.

14 Quoted in Dominik Wujastyk, *The Roots of Ayurveda: Selections from Sanskrit Medical Writings* (London, 2003), p. 326.

15 Ibid.

16 Rajiv Rastogi and Devesh Rastogi, 'Fasting as a Curative Practice: Historical, Traditional, and Contemporary Perspective', in *Ayurvedic Science of Food and Nutrition*, ed. Sanjeev Rastogi (New York, 2016), p. 124.

17 Wujastyk, *Roots of Ayurveda*, p. 283.

18 Sebastian Pole, *Ayurvedic Medicine: The Principles of Traditional Practice* (London, 2013), pp. 31–2.

19 Shripathi Adiga, 'Concept and Canons of Fasting in Ayurveda', *Journal of Fasting and Health*, 1/1 (2013), p. 38.

20 Jessica B. Gross, enLIGHTened: *How I Lost 40 Pounds with a Yoga Mat, Fresh Pineapples, and a Beagle Pointer* (New York, 2012), p. 130.

21 Ibid., p. 131.

22 Ibid., p. 132.

23 Ibid., p. 133.

24 Wujastyk, *Roots of Ayurveda*, p. 326.

25 Ibid.

26 Ibid.

27 'Ayurvedic Medicine: An Introduction', U.S. Department of Health and Human Services, National Institutes of Health National Center for Complementary and Integrative Health, August 2008, p. 2.

28 This comes from the Hippocratic treatise on epidemics.

29 Galen, *On the Properties of Foodstuffs* (Cambridge, 2003), p. 48.

30 Quoted in William Edward Fitch, *Dietotherapy* (New York, 1918), p. 112.

31 Wesley D. Smith et al., *Hippocrates* (London, 1923), vol. I, p. 31.

32 Veronika E. Grimm, *From Feasting to Fasting, the Evolution of a Sin: Attitudes to Food in Late Antiquity* (London, 1996), p. 53.

33 For more on this shift see Chapter Two of Walter Vandereycken and Ron Van Deth, *From Fasting Saints to Anorexic Girls: The History of Self-Starvation* (London, 1996).

34 Luigi Cornaro, *The Discourses and Letters of Louis Cornaro on a Sober and Temperate Life* (New York, 1842), p. 12.

35 Ibid., p. 9.

36 Ibid., p. 10.

37 Ibid., p. 16.

38 Klaus Bergdolt, *Wellbeing: A Cultural History of Healthy Living* (Cambridge, 2008), p. 184.

39 Cornaro, *Discourses and Letters*, p. 33.

40 Ibid.

41 Ibid., p. 27.

42 Ibid., p. 55.

43 Christoph Wilhelm Hufeland, *Hufeland's Art of Prolonging Life* (Boston, MA, 1854), p. 34.

44 Ibid., pp. 35–6.

45 Nathan Belofsky, *Strange Medicine: A Shocking History of Real Medical Practices Through the Ages* (New York, 2013), p. 88.

46 Avinash Sharma, *We Lived for the Body: Natural Medicine and Public Health in Imperial Germany* (DeKalb, IL, 2014), pp. 20–24.

47 For more information on Jennings see Natural Hygiene Press, *The Greatest Health Discovery: Natural Hygiene and It's* [sic] *Evolution Past, Present and Future* (Chicago, IL, 1972), pp. 33–8.

48 Quoted in Henry S. Tanner, *The Fasting Story* (Pomeroy, WA, 1956), p. 130.

49 Susan E. Cayleff, *Nature's Path: A History of Naturopathic Healing in America* (Baltimore, MD, 2016), p. 40.

50 Ibid., p. 32.

51 Quoted ibid., p. 119.

52 Quoted in Hereward Carrington, *Vitality, Fasting and Nutrition: A Physiological Study of the Curative Power of Fasting, Together with a New Theory of the Relation of Food to Human Vitality* (New York, 1908), p. 539.

53 Hillel Schwartz, *Never Satisfied: A Cultural History of Diets, Fantasies and Fat* (New York, 1986), p. 119.

54 Robert Alexander Gunn, *Forty Days Without Food! A Biography of Henry S. Tanner, MD, Including a Complete and Accurate History of His Wonderful Fasts* (New York, 1880), p. 12.

55 Tanner, *Fasting Story*, p. 84.

56 Gunn, *Forty Days Without Food!*, p. 17.

57 Ibid., p. 45.

58 Ibid., p. 78.

59 Ibid., p. 88.

60 Vandereycken and Deth, *Fasting Saints to Anorexic Girls*, p. 110.

61 'Gaining Health Through Fasting: What Some of the Followers of the Latest Fad Have Experienced in Seeking a Cure', *New York Times* (12 June 1910).

62 'Fasting as a Cure for Rheumatism: Time Required from 15 to 35 Days, Says the Founder of New Health Cult', *New York Times*, 12 April 1908, available at www.nytimes.com, accessed 3 August 2022.

63 Arnold Ehret, *Arnold Ehret's Mucusless-Diet Healing System: A Complete Course for Those Who Desire to Learn How to Control Their Health* (Beaumont, CA, 1953), pp. 44–5. Runaway white blood cell formation Ehret believed also to be the reason for Caucasians' white skin, a trait he considered wholly unnatural.

64 Norman W. Walker, *Pure and Simple Natural Weight Control* (Phoenix, AZ, 1981), p. 72.

65 Matthew C. L. Phillips, 'Fasting as a Therapy in Neurological Disease', *Nutrients*, XI/10 (2019), p. 3.
66 Dave Williams, *The Miracle Results of Fasting: Discover the Amazing Benefits in Your Spirit, Soul, and Body* (Tulsa, OK, 2005), p. 17.

4 SEEING LESS OF YOU: THE PROMISE OF FASTING FOR WEIGHT LOSS

1 Vance Thompson, *Eat and Grow Thin: The Mahdah Menus* (New York, 1914), p. 3.
2 'After Long Diet, He Dislikes Food', *The Sun* (18 July 1966), p. A3.
3 Ibid.
4 Jon Brady, 'The Tale of Angus Barbieri Who Fasted for More Than a Year – and Lost 21 Stone', *Evening Telegraph*, www.eveningtelegraph.co.uk, 12 November 2016.
5 Quoted in Gary Taubes, *Good Calories, Bad Calories: Challenging the Conventional Wisdom on Diet, Weight Control, and Disease* (New York, 2007), p. 258.
6 W. L. Bloom, 'Fasting as an Introduction to the Treatment of Obesity', *Metabolism: Clinical and Experimental*, VIII/3 (1959), p. 215.
7 Ibid.
8 Ibid., pp. 216–19.
9 Quoted in Taubes, *Good Calories*, p. 341.
10 Quoted ibid.
11 Ancel Keys, *The Biology of Human Starvation* (Minneapolis, MN, 1950), p. 507.
12 Victoria M., Gershuni, Stephanie L. Yan and Valentina Medici, 'Nutritional Ketosis for Weight Management and Reversal of Metabolic Syndrome', *Current Nutrition Reports*, VII (2018), p. 2.
13 John R. Butterly and Jack Shepherd, *Hunger: The Biology and Politics of Starvation* (Hanover, NH, 2010), pp. 93–4. The brain can go from feasting on some 150 grams (5 oz) of glucose a day to deriving about 65 per cent of its energy needs from ketones.
14 DeathNote55, 'Keto Removed My Appetite, It's So Strange', Reddit, February 2021, at www.reddit.com, accessed 7 May 2021.
15 Ibid.

16 Sarah E. Deemer, Catia Martins and Eric P. Plaisance, 'Impact of Ketosis on Appetite Regulation – A Review', *Nutrition Research*, LXXVII (2020), p. 8.

17 Antonio Paoli et al., 'Beyond Weight Loss: A Review of the Therapeutic Uses of Very-Low-Carbohydrate (Ketogenic) Diets', *European Journal of Clinical Nutrition*, LXVII/8 (2013), p. 2097.

18 Gershuni, Yan and Medici, 'Nutritional Ketosis', pp. 4–6.

19 Frank A. Evans, 'The Treatment of Obesity with Low Caloric Diets', *Journal of the American Medical Association*, XCVII/15 (1931), p. 1064.

20 People on ketogenic diets ought to consume no more than 50 grams of carbohydrates a day.

21 James J. Short, 'Extreme Obesity Followed by Therapeutic Reduction of Two Hundred and Thirty-Nine Pounds', *Journal of the American Medical Association*, CXI/24 (1938), p. 2196.

22 E. S. Garnett et al., 'Gross Fragmentation of Cardiac Myofibrils After Therapeutic Starvation for Obesity', *The Lancet*, CCXCIII/7601 (1969), p. 914.

23 Ibid., p. 916.

24 Ibid.

25 Ernst J. Drenick et al., 'Prolonged Starvation as Treatment for Severe Obesity', *Journal of the American Medical Association*, CLXXXVII/2 (1964), p. 144.

26 Ibid.

27 Ibid., p. 100.

28 Robert Levey, 'Fasting – The Ultimate Diet', *Boston Globe* (21 December 1975), p. B1.

29 Michael Goodwin, 'The Fastest Diet?', *New York Times* (15 August 1976), p. 173. Mt Sinai's fasting programme realized instant popularity. In addition to the four hundred individuals who participated, another 2,000 would-be fasters joined a waiting list.

30 Robert Linn and Sandra Lee Stuart, *The Last Chance Diet* (Des Plaines, IL, 1977), p. xii.

31 Nadine Brozan, 'The Liquid Protein Diet Controversy', *New York Times* (18 May 1977), p. 50.

32 Richard D. Lyons, 'FDA Warns Dieters About Liquid Protein', *New York Times* (10 November 1977), p. 1.

33 Ibid.

34 'Author of "The Last Chance Diet" Found Negligent', UPI,
   23 October 1981, www.upi.com, accessed 4 August 2022.
35 'Modified Fasting Helps in Treating Obesity', *Atlanta Daily World*
   (4 December 1986), p. 4.
36 Quoted in 'Oprah's Top 20 Moments', October 2005,
   www.oprah.com, accessed 4 August 2022.
37 A. M. Johnstone, 'Fasting – The Ultimate Diet?', *Obesity Reviews:
   An Official Journal of the International Association for the Study
   of Obesity*, VIII/3 (2007), p. 211.
38 Niki S. Papavramidou, Spiros T. Papavramidis and Helen
   Christopoulou-Aletra, 'Galen on Obesity: Etiology, Effects,
   and Treatment', *World Journal of Surgery*, XXVIII/6 (2004),
   pp. 632–3.
39 Ibid.
40 Quoted in Louise Foxcroft, *Calories and Corsets: A History of
   Dieting Over 2,000 Years* (London, 2013), p. 20.
41 Ken Albala, 'Weight Loss in the Age of Reason', in *Cultures of
   the Abdomen: Diet, Digestion and Fat in the Modern World*, ed.
   Christopher E. Forth and Ana Carden-Coyne (New York, 2005),
   pp. 170–71.
42 Ibid., p. 178.
43 Ibid., pp. 176–7.
44 Quoted in Lucia Dacome, 'Useless and Pernicious Matter:
   Corpulence in Eighteenth-Century England', in *Cultures of the
   Abdomen*, ed. Forth and Carden-Coyne, p. 186.
45 Thomas Short, *A Discourse Concerning the Causes and Effects
   of Corpulency* (London, 1728), p. 53.
46 Ibid., p. 9.
47 Sander L. Gilman, *Diets and Dieting: A Cultural Encyclopedia*
   (New York, 2009), p. 229.
48 James Boswell, *The Life of Samuel Johnson* (London, 1900),
   vol. II, p. 447.
49 James Boswell, *The Life of Samuel Johnson* (London, 1884),
   vol. III, p. 310.
50 Quoted in Foxcroft, *Calories and Corsets*, p. 20.
51 Hillel Schwartz, *Never Satisfied: A Cultural History of Diets,
   Fantasies, and Fat* (New York, 1986), p. 12.
52 Quoted ibid., p. 13.
53 Ibid., p. 14.

54 Quoted ibid., p. 13.
55 Alfred William Moore, *Corpulency* (London, 1857), p. 15.
56 Ibid., p. 10.
57 Ibid., p. 8.
58 Edward Hooker Dewey, *The No-Breakfast Plan and the Fasting-Cure* (Meadville, PA, 1900), pp. 28–9.
59 Ibid., p. 63.
60 Quoted in Bernarr Macfadden and Felix Oswald, *Macfadden's Fasting, Hydropathy and Exercise* (London, 1903), p. 28.
61 Dewey, *No-Breakfast Plan*, p. 64.
62 James Whorton, *Crusaders for Fitness: The History of American Health Reformers* (Princeton, NJ, 1982), p. 266.
63 Dewey, *No-Breakfast Plan*, p. 75.
64 Vanessa Heggie, 'Diets, Fads, and the Methods of Science', *The Guardian*, www.theguardian.com, 8 January 2013.
65 'Food and Feeding', *British Medical Journal*, I/2563 (1910), p. 388.
66 Antoine Aoun, 'The Safety and Efficacy of Intermittent Fasting for Weight Loss', *Nutrition Today*, LV/6 (2020), p. 271.
67 Guolin Li et al., 'Intermittent Fasting Promotes White Adipose Browning and Decreases Obesity by Shaping the Gut Microbiota', *Cell Metabolism*, XXVI/5 (2017), p. 672.
68 Mark E. Smyers et al., 'Enhanced Weight and Fat Loss from Long-Term Intermittent Fasting in Obesity-Prone, Low-Fitness Rats', *Physiology and Behavior*, CCXXX/10 (2021), p. 9.
69 Peter Bowes, 'Intermittent Fasting: The Good Things It Did to My Body', BBC News, www.bbc.co.uk, 3 January 2014.
70 Ibid.
71 Zoe Williams, 'Fit in My 40s: Will Intermittent Fasting Boost My Energy Levels?', *The Guardian*, www.theguardian.com, 16 January 2021.
72 Valter D. Longo and Satchidananda Panda, 'Fasting, Circadian Rhythms, and Time-Restricted Feeding in Healthy Lifespan', *Cell Metabolism*, XXIII/6 (2016), p. 1048.
73 Ibid., p. 1051.
74 'Intermittent Fasting: The Positive News Continues', Harvard Health Blog, 29 June 2018, www.health.harvard.edu, accessed 5 August 2022.

75 Aoun, 'Safety and Efficacy of Intermittent Fasting',
   p. 275.
76 Nicholas Bakalar, 'Fasting Offers No Special Weight Loss
   Benefits', *New York Times*, 3 May 2017, www.nytimes.com,
   accessed 5 August 2022.

5 THE WAGES OF THIN: THE PERILS OF FASTING FOR WEIGHT LOSS

1 Alon Altaras, 'What Can Be Learned from One of the First
   Known Eating Disorder Patients', *Haaretz*, www.haaretz.com,
   8 February 2022.
2 Quoted in Hilde Bruch, *Eating Disorders: Obesity,
   Anorexia Nervosa, and the Person Within* (New York, 1973),
   p. 219.
3 Ludwig Binswanger, 'The Case of Ellen West: An
   Anthropological–Clinical Study', in *Existence: A New Dimension
   in Psychiatry and Psychology*, ed. R. May, E. Angel and H. F.
   Ellenberger (New York, 1958), p. 239.
4 Ibid., p. 242.
5 Ibid., pp. 242–3, 248 and 249.
6 Ibid., p. 249.
7 Quoted in Bruch, *Eating Disorders*, p. 220.
8 Quoted ibid., p. 221.
9 Ibid., pp. 252–3.
10 Ibid., p. 255.
11 Ibid., p. 256.
12 Ibid.
13 Ibid.
14 Veronika Grimm, 'Fasting Women in Judaism and Christianity
   in Late Antiquity', in *Food in Antiquity*, ed. John Wilkins and
   David Harvey (Exeter, 1995), p. 236.
15 Walter Vandereycken and Ron Van Deth, *From Fasting Saints
   to Anorexic Girls: The History of Self-Starvation* (London, 1996),
   p. 218.
16 Ibid.
17 All quotes from Bruch, *Eating Disorders*, pp. 211–12.
18 Ibid., p. 285.
19 Ibid.

20 Ibid., p. 286.

21 J. R. Bemporad, 'Self-Starvation Through the Ages: Reflections on the Pre-History of Anorexia Nervosa', *International Journal of Eating Disorders*, XIX/3 (1996), pp. 228–9.

22 Vandereycken and Van Deth, *Fasting Saints to Anorexic Girls*, p. 124.

23 William Somerset Maugham, *Of Human Bondage* (New York, 1915), pp. 334–5.

24 William Withey Gull, *A Collection of the Published Writings of William Withey Gull* (London, 1894), pp. 305–7.

25 Ibid., p. 307.

26 Ibid., pp. 306–7.

27 Ibid., p. 311.

28 Ibid.

29 Vandereycken and Van Deth, *Fasting Saints to Anorexic Girls*, p. 163.

30 Regina C. Casper, 'The "Drive for Activity" and "Restlessness" in Anorexia Nervosa: Potential Pathways', *Journal of Affective Disorders*, XCII/1 (2006), pp. 99–107.

31 Vandereycken and Van Deth, *Fasting Saints to Anorexic Girls*, p. 163.

32 Ibid.

33 For more on these physicians, see Edward Stainbrook, 'Psychosomatic Medicine in the Nineteenth Century', *Psychosomatic Medicine*, XIV/3 (1952), pp. 211–27.

34 Vandereycken and Van Deth, *Fasting Saints to Anorexic Girls*, pp. 175–6.

35 Ibid., p. 182.

36 Ibid.

37 G. K. Ushakov, 'Anorexia Nervosa, in *Modern Perspectives in Adolescent Psychiatry*, 4th edn, ed. J. G. Howells (Edinburgh, 1971), pp. 277–8.

38 Vandereycken and Van Deth, *Fasting Saints to Anorexic Girls*, p. 237.

39 All quotes from L. Sprague de Camp, *Lovecraft: A Biography* (Garden City, NY, 1975), p. 362.

40 Quoted in Ali Pattillo, 'Intermittent Fasting: A Popular Diet with Serious Psychological Risks', *Inverse*, www.inverse.com, 29 July 2019.

41 Eric Stice et al., 'Fasting Increases Risk for Onset of Binge Eating and Bulimic Pathology: A 5-Year Prospective Study', *Journal of Abnormal Psychology*, CXVII/4 (2008), p. 5.

42 Quoted in Pattillo, 'Intermittent Fasting'.

43 George Alexander, 'Brown Rice as a Way of Life', *New York Times* (12 March 1972), p. 90.

44 Sakurazawa Nyoiti, *You Are All Sanpaku* (New York, 1965), p. 94.

45 Ibid.

46 Ibid., p. 101.

47 Ibid., p. 20.

48 Ibid., p. 22.

49 Ibid., pp. 24–5.

50 Alexander, 'Brown Rice'.

51 Quoted ibid.

52 Ibid.

53 B. Gaborit et al., 'Ramadan Fasting with Diabetes: An Interview Study of Inpatients' and General Practitioners' Attitudes in the South of France', *Diabetes and Metabolism*, XXXVII/5 (2011), p. 400.

54 U.S. Centers for Disease Control and Prevention, 'Hyperthermia and Dehydration-Related Deaths Associated with Intentional Rapid Weight Loss in Three Collegiate Wrestlers – North Carolina, Wisconsin, and Michigan, November–December 1997', *Morbidity and Mortality Weekly Report*, XLVII/6 (1998), p. 824.

55 'Killed by Dieting', *Auckland Star* (7 January 1927), p. 12.

56 Steven Mintz and Susan Kellogg, *Domestic Revolutions: A Social History of American Family Life* (New York, 1988), p. 182.

57 Oliver Goldsmith, *The Vicar of Wakefield* (London, 1897), p. 13.

58 Stephanie Coontz, *The Social Origins of Private Life: A History of American Families, 1600–1900* (London, 1988), p. 182.

59 Mintz and Kellogg, *Domestic Revolutions*, p. 23.

60 Clotaire Rapaille, *The Culture Code: An Ingenious Way to Understand Why People Around the World Buy and Live as They Do* (New York, 2006), p. 111.

61 Ibid., p. 103.

62 Ibid.

63 Ibid.

64 Georg Simmel, *Simmel on Culture: Selected Writings* (London, 1997), p. 130.

65 Elaine N. McIntosh, *American Food Habits in Historical Perspective* (Westport, CT, 1995), p. 152.

66 'Intermittent Fasting: The Positive News Continues', Harvard Health Blog, 29 June 2018, www.health.harvard.edu, accessed 6 August 2022.

67 E. A. Chowdhury et al., 'Effect of Extended Morning Fasting upon Ad Libitum Lunch Intake and Associated Metabolic and Hormonal Responses in Obese Adults', *International Journal of Obesity*, XL/2 (2016), p. 308.

EPILOGUE: OF APPS AND APPETITE – THE FUTURE OF FASTING

1 MyFast, at myfasttracker.com, accessed 15 March 2021.

2 Olivia Solon, 'The Silicon Valley Execs Who Don't Eat for Days: "It's Not Dieting, It's Biohacking"', *The Guardian*, www.theguardian.com, 4 September 2017.

3 WeFast Slack channel, accessed 30 August 2021.

4 Ibid.

5 'Our 5 Day Extended Fasting Experience', Have Butter Will Travel, 19 August 2019, www.havebutterwilltravel.com, accessed 10 August 2022.

6 Simply Quinoa, 'My 3-Day Juice Cleanse Experience', YouTube, www.youtube.com, accessed 10 August 2022.

7 Michael Baumgarthuber, personal communication, 17 August 2019.

8 Sura Detox, at www.suradetox.co.uk, accessed 30 August 2021.

9 Tonya Williams Bradford, Sonya A. Grier and Geraldine Rosa Henderson, 'Weight Loss Through Virtual Support Communities: A Role for Identity-Based Motivation in Public Commitment', *Journal of Interactive Marketing*, XL/1 (2017), pp. 9–23.

10 Gemma Flores Mateo et al., 'Mobile Phone Apps to Promote Weight Loss and Increase Physical Activity: A Systematic Review and Meta-Analysis', *Journal of Medical Internet Research*, XVII/11 (2015).

11 Jumana Antoun et al., 'The Effectiveness of Combining Nonmobile Interventions with the Use of Smartphone Apps with Various Features for Weight Loss: Systematic Review and Meta-Analysis', *JMIR mHealth and uHealth*, X/4 (2022).

SELECT BIBLIOGRAPHY

Albala, Ken, 'Weight Loss in the Age of Reason', in *Cultures of the Abdomen: Diet, Digestion and Fat in the Modern World*, ed. Christopher E. Forth and Ana Carden-Coyne (New York, 2005)

Bergdolt, Klaus, *Wellbeing: A Cultural History of Healthy Living* (Cambridge, 2008)

Bruch, Hilde, *Eating Disorders: Obesity, Anorexia Nervosa, and the Person Within* (New York, 1973)

Butterly, John R., and Jack Shepherd, *Hunger: The Biology and Politics of Starvation* (Hanover, NH, 2010)

Cayleff, Susan E., *Nature's Path: A History of Naturopathic Healing in America* (Baltimore, MD, 2016)

Cornaro, Luigi, *The Discourses and Letters of Louis Cornaro on a Sober and Temperate Life* (New York, 1842)

Dewey, Edward Hooker, *The No-Breakfast Plan and the Fasting-Cure* (Meadville, PA, 1900)

Gilman, Sander L., *Diets and Dieting: A Cultural Encyclopedia* (New York, 2009)

Hamsun, Knut, *Hunger* (New York, 1920)

Jotischky, Andrew, *A Hermit's Cookbook: Monks, Food and Fasting in the Middle Ages* (London, 2011)

Keys, Ancel, *The Biology of Human Starvation* (Minneapolis, MN, 1950)

Rapaille, Clotaire, *The Culture Code: An Ingenious Way to Understand Why People Around the World Buy and Live as They Do* (New York, 2006)

Russell, Sharman Apt, *Hunger: An Unnatural History* (New York, 2006)

Schwartz, Hillel, *Never Satisfied: A Cultural History of Diets, Fantasies, and Fat* (New York, 1986)

Sharma, Avinash, *We Lived for the Body: Natural Medicine and Public Health in Imperial Germany* (DeKalb, IL, 2014)

Taubes, Gary, *Good Calories, Bad Calories: Challenging the Conventional Wisdom on Diet, Weight Control, and Disease* (New York, 2007)

Vandereycken, Walter, and Ron Van Deth, *From Fasting Saints to Anorexic Girls: The History of Self-Starvation* (London, 1996)

Winick, Myron, *Hunger Disease: Studies by the Jewish Physicians in the Warsaw Ghetto* (New York, 1979)

Wujastyk, Dominik, *The Roots of Ayurveda: Selections from Sanskrit Medical Writings* (London, 2003)

ACKNOWLEDGEMENTS

I wish to thank my Opa and Oma, Josef and Hildegard Baumgarthuber, for introducing me to fasting and sound nutrition. Thanks also go to Erwin Montgomery for his help with the manuscript, and to everyone at Reaktion Books for their guidance and assistance, especially Michael Leaman. Finally, I'd like to thank the folks at Internet Archive, quite possibly one of the only good and idealistic things left on the Internet, for keeping many hard-to-find and out-of-print books accessible to the public.

INDEX